Practice Teaching in Healthcare

Practice Teaching in Healthcare

Neil Gopee

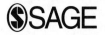

Los Angeles | London | New Delhi
Singapore | Washington DC

© Neil Gopee 2010

First published 2010

SAGE Publications Ltd
1 Oliver's Yard
55 City Road
London EC1Y 1SP

SAGE Publications Inc.
2455 Teller Road
Thousand Oaks, California 91320

SAGE Publications India Pvt Ltd
B 1/I 1 Mohan Cooperative Industrial Area
Mathura Road
New Delhi 110 044

SAGE Publications Asia-Pacific Pte Ltd
33 Pekin Street #02-01
Far East Square
Singapore 048763

Library of Congress Control Number: 2009931948

British Library Cataloguing in Publication data

A catalogue record for this book is available from
the British Library

ISBN 978-1-84860-134-5
ISBN 978-1-84860-135-2

Typeset by C&M Digitals (P) Ltd, Chennai, India
Printed in Great Britain by MPG Books Group, Bodmin, Cornwall
Printed on paper from sustainable resources

Mixed Sources
Product group from well-managed
forests and other controlled sources
www.fsc.org Cert no. SA-COC-1565
© 1996 Forest Stewardship Council

Contents

List of Boxes

List of Figures

List of Tables

Foreword

As a professor of nursing and as a lecturer, I can recall my move from being a charge nurse in care of the elderly, to that of an unqualified nurse teacher. My new role entailed supporting, teaching and assessing students in practice – and I was the only one. This was a huge change and challenge for me, and required me drawing on existing, as well as new, knowledge and skills. Yes, I know, I was able to talk to my clinical teacher and nurse teacher colleagues, but I would have really benefited from access to a book such as *Practice Teaching in Healthcare*. This is an important and timely publication for practice teachers – there is a paucity of information to guide and inform these practitioners – Neil Gopee's book fills this gap, providing an excellent resource for those supporting students in practice.

The divide between what is taught in the academy and what is performed in practice has been debated, and suggestions on the best way to facilitate practice-based teaching well documented. Those of us in healthcare work in an environment of frequent and rapid change, where we need to have the skills to identify an issue, access and retrieve information, assess the quality of this information, and apply this in our practice. Gopee's book will smooth the progress of this for practitioners embarking on the journey to become practice teachers.

This book takes the policy 'Standards to Support Learning and Assessment in Practice' (NMC, 2008) and translates it into practice – in order that practice teachers can ask the question 'How do I develop my students practice?' Gopee facilitates this by using the eight domains from the Nursing and Midwifery Council as a framework (NMC, 2008), where each domain is a chapter. He then encourages the practitioner to take the theories, frameworks and concepts highlighted and to apply them to their practice area. This helps to close a loop by providing a rationale, linking theory with practice, and provides the practice teacher (and their students) with the opportunity to integrate an academic dimension into their everyday practice (i.e. evidence-based practice).

This book provides the practitioner with the opportunity to explore issues of their choice, pertinent to their practice, and ask questions such as 'How can I contribute to the learning experience of this student?'; 'How do I enrich my practice with knowledge from evidence?'; or 'How does my practice contribute the learning community?' Gopee has drawn on a range of current and seminal evidence to support each chapter, and the use of case studies helps the reader make sense as well as see how they might apply a theory to their area of practice. From a student perspective, it is much easier to work with someone who is not only a skilled practitioner, but someone who is not afraid to provoke and challenge the student's thoughts and perspectives – a quizzical companion.

I first became aware of Neil Gopee through his teaching and research, particularly in the area of mentoring. Having read his work, I have also drawn on his expertise by inviting him to contribute to a book I was editing on study skills for nurses and midwives (Gopee, 2010 in Maslin-Prothero). It is good to see him continuing to share this specialist knowledge and expertise, and applying it to the important art of teaching in practice. This text will help the reader make sense of policy, how it influences their role, as well as providing them with the tools to inspire and develop students.

Sian Maslin-Prothero RN, Cert Ed, PhD, MSc, DipN
Professor of Nursing and Dean of the Graduate School
University of Keele, Staffordshire, United Kingdom

References

Gopee N. (2010) 'Developing a portfolio' In: Maslin-Prothero S. E. (ed). *Bailliere's Study Skills for Nurses and Midwives* 4th edition. London, Bailliere Tindall, Chapter 15.

Nursing and Midwifery Council (NMC) (2008) *Standards to Support Learning and Assessment in Practice*. London, NMC.

Acknowledgements

I would like to thank Zoe Elliott-Fawcett, Alison Poyner and Emma Patterson at SAGE Publications for the support and constructive comments provided; and my wonderful daughters Neeta, Sheila and Hema for their ongoing support with these ventures

Abbreviations

AANPE	Association of Advanced Nursing Practice Educators
ALS	action learning sets
ANP	advanced nurse practitioner
AP(E)L	accreditation of prior (experiential) learning
CAIPE	Centre for Advancement of Interprofessional Education
CBT	cognitive behaviour therapy
CFP	common foundation programme
CHRE	Council for Healthcare Regulatory Excellence
CNS	clinical nurse specialist
CPD	continuing professional development
CPT	community practice teacher
DH	Department of Health
EBP	evidence-based practice
EBHC	evidence-based healthcare
ENB	English National Board for Nursing, Midwifery and Health Visiting
EWS	early warning system
EWTD	European Working Time Directive
GMC	General Medical Council
HEI	higher education institute
HPC	Health Professions Council
ICN	International Council for Nurses
IPE	interprofessional education
MMC	Modernising Medical Careers
NCIHE	National Committee of Inquiry into Higher Education
NMC	Nursing and Midwifery Council
NHS KSF	NHS Knowledge and Skills Framework
NICE	National Institute for Health and Clinical Excellence
NSF	National Service Frameworks
PBL	problem-based learning
PDP	personal development plans
PEF	practice education facilitator
PESTLE	political, economic, social, technological, legal and ethical
QAA	Quality Assurance Agency for Higher Education
RCN	Royal College of Nursing
RCT	ramdomised controlled trial
SCPHN	specialist community public health nurse
SLT	social learning theory
SPQ	specialist practice qualification

SWOT	strengths, weakness, opportunities and threats
UKCC	United Kingdom Central Council for Nursing, Midwifery and Health Visiting
WBL	work-based learning

Introduction

Welcome to this book on the relatively novel practice teacher role. This introduction to the book presents the rationale, scope and aims of the book, the structure of the essential components addressed and how to use the book.

The rationale, scope and aims of this book

This book on practice teaching explores the knowledge and skills required for supporting learning, and for assessing the knowledge and competence of students on specialist and advanced practice programmes. The role is currently predominantly for nurses but the principles and theories underpinning competent fulfilment of such roles are transferable and can be applied directly to other healthcare and social-care professionals learning support roles for learning beyond initial registration. The practice teacher's role is defined by the criteria, competencies and educational preparation requirements for the role as delineated by the Nursing and Midwifery Council [NMC] (2008a).

Practice teaching as a concept has prevailed since 2005 in an NMC circular, when it was instituted specifically for the facilitation of learning and the assessment of the competence of qualified nurses on specialist and advanced practice educational-preparation programmes. There is a paucity of textbooks available to facilitate practice teachers' role development, hence this textbook, which examines in detail the knowledge and competence required by healthcare professionals to fulfil this role effectively. The role incorporates consideration of relevant research, policy directives and potential issues.

Specific areas of knowledge and competence have been identified by the NMC (2008a) under eight domains, an overall descriptor or competence for each domain, and a number of outcomes or competencies. The domains are: establishing effective working relationships, facilitation of learning, assessment and accountability, evaluation of learning, creating an environment for learning, context of practice, evidence-based practice and leadership. The aim of this textbook is to examine the knowledge and competence required to fulfil the practice teacher role by critically evaluating and building on the concepts and theories inherent within the eight domains, and related outcomes.

The practice teacher's main function in the supervision of learning and the assessment of competence of students on specialist or advanced practice courses is one that has emerged to meet a provision that is recognised by healthcare professionals, healthcare trusts and the NMC. The role incorporates signing-off proficiency for qualified healthcare professionals on various post-qualifying courses, and also for pre-registration students on their final practice placement.

Initially the practice teaching role has been required predominantly for the supervision and assessment of students on specialist community public health nursing (SCPHN) courses, and it looks likely to become a requirement for supervising students on all clinical nurse specialist (CNS) and advanced nurse practitioner (ANP) courses. Consequently, there will be a need for more practice teachers in various specialisms in healthcare trusts in forthcoming years, and several higher education institutions (HEI) already offer programmes to meet this need.

Practice teaching is a component of the NMC's (2008a) developmental framework to support learning and assessment in practice, and is intercalated between the mentor and NMC approved teacher roles. Practice teaching therefore builds on healthcare professionals' existing expertise in supporting learning as a registrant and mentor by recognising their expertise, and enabling them to further develop and advance their knowledge and competence for supporting students on specialist practice qualifications (SPQ) and ANP courses. Students on SPQ and ANP courses, be it in acute, primary or continuing care, require a detailed and deep understanding of specific clinical interventions, and this book endeavours to enable the practice teacher to facilitate the acquisition of the necessary specialist or advanced clinical skills and knowledge.

Healthcare professionals will have met the NMC's outcomes for mentors through either a mentor educational preparation programme or through the accreditation of prior (experiential) learning (AP[E]L). Although not research-proven, it appears that the usual single module (approximately 200 hours of student effort) mentor course does not adequately equip the mentor to supervise and assess students on specialist or advanced practice courses. The previous corresponding role towards students on community care courses was entitled 'community practice teacher' (CPT) (and later to some extent a practice teacher role for supervising students on community psychiatric nursing courses), and the educational preparation for these roles was generally HEI-based.

The structure of this book

The book achieves the above-mentioned aims by examining specific concepts that are inherent within the NMC's eight domains and outcomes, which are addressed as eight chapters, the first one of which examines the reasons, aims and scope of practice teaching, and the current position with specialist and advanced practice. Subsequent chapters examine:

- the management of inter-professional relationships in healthcare
- facilitating learning of generic, specialist and advanced clinical practice skills
- assessing specialist and advanced practice knowledge and competence
- the practice teacher's role in evidence-based practice and practice development
- the practice teacher's accountability
- practice teaching and leadership
- contemporary issues and further developments in practice teaching in healthcare and social-care professions, and continuing professional development (CPD) for practice teachers.

In brief detail, therefore, Chapter 1 – 'The Scope of the Practice Teacher Role' – begins by exploring in detail the rationales for the practice teacher role, and defines and distinguishes it from related teaching roles such as practice education facilitators (PEF) (or practice educators), mentors, ANPs, CNSs and consultant healthcare professionals. This is followed by an examination of specialist and advanced practice roles, and the diverse developments in this area. National and international standards for specialist and advanced practice are explored, along with current debates and research, which are inherent components of these concepts. The chapter then explores educational preparation programmes for both specialist and advanced practice, and practice teacher roles.

Chapter 2 – 'Establishing and Managing Effective Working Relationships as a Practice Teacher' – examines the reasons for cultivating working relationships in the supervision of learning specifically in relation to practice teaching. It also explores the nature and dynamics of professional and inter-professional relationships between healthcare professionals and their students, and with patients and service users, and the systematic ways in which they are formed, maintained and managed. Potential difficulties in establishing effective working relationships are also examined, and how they can be averted or resolved.

Chapter 3 – 'Facilitating Learning of Specialist and Advanced Clinical Practice' – focuses on the facilitation of learning for students on specialist and advanced practice courses, and those approaching completion of their pre-registration programmes. It explores the distinction between teaching and the facilitation of learning, and the most significant contemporary concepts and models of teaching and learning. The practice teacher's role in the facilitation of learning of generic and specialist/advanced practice knowledge and competence is discussed, including the supervision of practice learning for students on SPQ and ANP programmes, as well as potential obstacles to this. Finally, the chapter takes a critical look at the practice teacher's role in supporting learning in academic environments, and student learning at different academic levels.

Chapter 4 – 'The Practice Teacher, Evidence-based Practice and Practice Development' – centres on the practice teacher as an evidence-based practitioner in the context of specialist and advanced practice, and as a practice developer. Being a researcher, an innovator and a 'nurse entrepreneur' are inherent concepts, and activities that incorporate managing change and innovations, as well as disseminating innovative clinical practices.

The focus of Chapter 5 – 'Assessing Specialist and Advanced practice Knowledge and Competence' – is on the assessment of the knowledge and competence of healthcare professionals on specialist and advanced practice courses. The chapter begins by exploring the general nature of assessments, and incorporates assessing the professional knowledge and competence of students on SPQ and ANP programmes, as well as finalist pre-registration students. Assessment at different academic levels utilising assessment strategies and frameworks is explored, together with research on the assessment of competencies and service-user involvement in assessments. Safe and effective practice forms the focus of assessments, along with maintaining academic and professional standards.

Chapter 6 – 'The Practice Teacher's Accountability' – starts by exploring the reasons for scrutinising the practice teacher's accountability and responsibilities in facilitating learning and assessment. It therefore examines the nature of accountability, and the parameters of the practice teacher's accountability, accountability in the assessment of knowledge and competence, ways of monitoring students' progress, how to manage underachievement in supervisees and the implications of pass/fail decisions, together with the ethical implications of these.

In Chapter 7 – Practice Teaching and Leadership – how the practice teacher can exercise leadership is analysed. Definitions and the scope of the concept of leadership, and the theories and framework of effective leadership, are addressed, together with the practice teacher's leadership in managing the challenges of supporting learning, such as the competing demands of their clinical practice, education, administrative and other roles.

Theory–practice integration and forward planning are seen as essential leadership capabilities, as is the practice teacher's leadership in the education and assessment of SPQ, ANP and pre-registration students, as well as their leadership in evaluating the effectiveness of practice teaching.

As a recently instituted concept, practice teaching will gradually evolve within different clinical specialisms. Further developments on practice teaching are also anticipated as the NMC's standards for learning and assessment in practice are embedded and the arising issues are redressed. Chapter 8 – 'Issues and Further Developments in Facilitating the Acquisition of Specialist and Advanced Practice Skills' – explores these likely developments and issues that might surface in both practice teaching, and specialist and advanced practice, including the career structure of specialist and advanced practitioners, quality indicators for their clinical activities, and educational preparation and CPD for practice teachers. How these issues can be anticipated and managed will be examined.

All major concepts are looked at against the backdrop of the key questions: what the concept is about, why practice teachers need to know about it, how it is done, and any issues and developments. The components addressed cross-reference the literature on teaching in the healthcare professions throughout.

As for special features, each chapter opens with an introduction identifying the focus of the chapter, and chapter outcomes, and concludes with a chapter summary that identifies the areas addressed. Boxes, tables and figures are included as illustrations where appropriate. The text also includes action points and some case studies, with the former designed to engage the reader in critical thinking and problem solving, and for reflecting on the application of relevant knowledge to practice teacher work.

How to use this book

Practice Teaching in Healthcare is different from all other textbooks on the subject area, in that it is specifically for practice teachers supervising students on specialist and advanced practice courses, and it therefore examines inherent concepts in the context of current knowledge in the field, and how they apply to the practice teacher role, as well as to developments and issues. It is anticipated that this book will be a core textbook for nurses and midwives on practice teacher programmes, and a guide for other healthcare and social-care professionals with the practice teacher role, as the principles and practices explored are largely the same and therefore apply to all health and related professions.

However, the textbook is not necessarily designed to be a manual or handbook (for practice teaching), which by implication can be prescriptive, but instead identifies and examines relevant theories, frameworks and concepts (and their application to practice), that constitute the practice teacher's armoury of knowledge and competence, and templates to become competent as a practice teacher.

I anticipate the book will be used by students on practice teacher courses. The NMC website identifies several universities as already approved to run the practice teacher course, and although it is thought that initially the uptake of the course might be slow as students on specialist and advanced practice courses are currently assessed by experienced mentors and by medical practitioners with appropriate skills. This book also provides a valuable update for previously qualified practice teachers, for example CPT and healthcare and social-care professionals supervising students on community psychiatric nursing and similar courses, for preceptors and aspiring teachers.

Furthermore, practice teacher educational preparation courses can form part of Master's in Education programmes, or those that encompass the achievement of NMC Advanced Practitioner competencies, and lead to awards such as an MSc in Advancing Practice.

1

The Scope of the Practice Teacher Role

Introduction

Having identified the rationales for this textbook, and its scope and structure, in the Introduction, Chapter 1 focuses on the reasons for, and the scope of, the practice teacher role. It therefore identifies developments in the educational preparation of healthcare professionals beyond the initial registration that led to the creation of this role, which is closely linked to developments in specialist and advanced practice. Its major focus is therefore on the facilitation of learning for qualified nurses on post-qualifying educational programmes at specialist and advanced practice levels, and thus also on the requirements of the NMC (2008a) in terms of standards and outcomes for practice teachers for supporting learning and assessment in practice.

Subsequent chapters explore establishing and managing inter-professional relationships, facilitating the learning of generic, specialist and advanced clinical practice skills, assessing specialist and advanced practice knowledge and competence, the practice teacher's role as evidence-based practitioner and practice developer, the practice teacher's accountability, practice teaching and leadership, and contemporary issues and further developments in practice teaching in nursing, and in healthcare and social care.

Chapter outcomes

On completion of this chapter you should be able to:

1 Enunciate a number of reasons for the practice teacher role, identify the scope, and the competence and outcomes for the role, distinguish between practice teacher and similar roles, and then identify the criteria for effective implementation of the role.
2 Identify the factors that are driving the development of specialist and advanced practice roles, including national policies and research on the effectiveness of these roles, and how these developments interface with post-qualifying career frameworks for healthcare practitioners.
3 Critically analyse the nature of contemporary specialist and advanced practice roles, taking into consideration the NMC's standpoint on specialist practice qualifications, and review the implementation of standards for advanced nursing practice.
4 Evaluate the educational preparation for specialist and advanced practice roles, and for the practice teacher role.

Why practice teaching?

The practice teacher role was identified by the NMC (2005a), and its scope depicted in detail in 2006 in the first edition of *Standards to Support Learning and Assessment in Practice,* as a role that is required to support practice-based learning for students on specialist and advanced practice programmes. The first section of this chapter explores the nature and requirements of the practice teacher role, the reasons for creating this new role, and the criteria and scope of this role.

What is this new role and why?

The NMC (2008a) indicates that a practice teacher is a registrant who is normally already a qualified, and therefore competent, mentor, and who has received further educational preparation to gain the knowledge and competence required to meet the NMC's outcomes for the practice teacher role. It indicates that a practice teacher is 'A registrant who has gained knowledge, skills and competence in both their specialist area of practice and in their teaching role, meeting the outcomes of stage 3, and who facilitates learning, supervises and assesses students in a practice setting' (NMC, 2008a: 45). The mentor course generally does not encompass preparation for supervision of students on SPQ and ANP programmes adequately, predominantly because it is completed in a relatively short period of time.

Practice teachers are therefore CNSs or ANPs who have successfully completed an additional programme of study in the facilitation of learning and assessment of the clinical competence of students on learning beyond initial registration courses, including in signing-off the proficiency of pre-registration students. They also have to fulfil other job requirements as determined by the employing healthcare trust.

Action point 1.1 – Why the practice teacher role?

Other than the NMC's requirement for the practice teacher role, think of other reasons from your own professional experience why this role might be required.

In community nursing, the predecessors to the practice teacher role were such roles as the CPT, and supervisors of trainee community psychiatric nurses. The educational preparation for the CPT role generally comprised a one-year-long part-time course based in HEIs. The role was overlooked in the United Kingdom Central Council for Nursing, Midwifery and Health Visiting's (UKCC) (2000) *Preparation of Teachers of Nursing and Midwifery* document. Educational preparation of both the CPT course and the predecessor of the mentor course were of longer duration than most of the current practice teacher and mentor courses.

Another reason for this role is that specialist and advanced practice roles and titles are currently diverse and ill defined, and employees and appointees can decide locally as to the precise nature of these roles. There is of course a fair amount of research on specialist and advanced practice roles already, as well as recent national guidelines that incorporate the competencies required for these roles.

The NMC (2008a) indicates that the purposes of the practice teacher role in supporting learning in practice are to:

- Provide support and guidance to the student when learning new skills, applying new knowledge and transferring existing knowledge and competence to a new context of practice.
- Act as a resource to the student to facilitate learning and professional growth for specialist practice.
- Manage the student's learning in practice in order to ensure public protection.
- Directly observe the student's practice, or use indirect observation where appropriate, to ensure that NMC defined outcomes and competencies are met.

Criteria for the practice teacher role

Nurses' professional activities can generally be categorised into four components, namely clinical practice, the organisation and management of care, educating and research. *The NHS Knowledge and Skills Framework (NHS KSF)* (Department of Health [DH], 2004a) identifies six groups of activities for NHS posts, which are referred to as core dimensions, 24 specific dimensions that apply to particular but not all groups of posts in the NHS, and for each dimension there are a number of 'level descriptors' and several 'indicators'. The core dimensions are: (i) communication, (ii) personal and people development, (iii) health, safety and security, (iv) service improvement, (v) quality, and (vi) equality and diversity. The core dimension personal and people development, and the specific dimension 'Learning and development', are the categories that detail the competencies required for supporting learning roles, such as that of practice teacher. As to who can be a practice teacher, the NMC (2008a) is quite clear about who can adopt this role and title, the criteria for which are identified in Box 1.1.

Box 1.1   Criteria for the practice teacher role

Nurses who intend to take on the role of practice teacher, and who will be assessing the student's fitness for practice, must fulfil the following criteria:

- Be registered in the same part of the register, i.e. SCPHN, and from the same field of practice, e.g. school nursing, health visiting or occupational-health nursing (or relevant SPQ where this is a local requirement), as the student they are to assess.
- Have developed their own knowledge, skills and competence beyond registration, i.e. registered and worked for at least two years, and gained additional qualifications that will support students in SCPHN, or SPQ where this is a local requirement.
- Have successfully completed an NMC approved practice teacher preparation programme or a comparable HEI programme that addresses the NMC practice teacher requirements. They will normally have previously met the NMC outcomes for mentors and gained experience in this role.

- Have the abilities to design, deliver and assess programmes of learning in clinical settings for a range of students and learners in their field of practice.
- Be able to support learning in an interprofessional environment by supporting a range of learning opportunities within their level of practice and specialist expertise.
- Be able to use agreed criteria for cross-professional assessment and supervise mentors and other healthcare professionals using such criteria.
- Be able to make judgements about the competence/proficiency of NMC students, for registration on the same part of the register, and be accountable for such decisions.
- Be able to provide leadership to all those involved in supporting learning and assessing in practice for NMC students – enabling effective learning environments to be developed.

Source: NMC, 2008a

The scope of practice teaching

The scope of the practice teacher role is firmly founded on the knowledge and competence required to fulfil this role effectively. However, learning for students on specialist and advanced practice educational preparation programmes is supported by a range of healthcare and social-care expert clinicians, often in more senior clinical roles, and experienced in the facilitation of learning for healthcare profession students, and other more junior qualified colleagues.

The practice teaching role was defined earlier, but there are various overlapping and related roles, and this section endeavours to disentangle the anticipated similarities, differences and overlaps between them. (Some of these roles are defined in the Glossary at the back of this book.) Such roles include (NMC-approved) teacher, mentor, learning supervisor, sign-off mentor, PEF and inter-professional learning facilitators; and also clinical nurse specialists, AHP consultants (e.g. consultant physiotherapist) and autonomous practitioners, such as nurses who run nurse-led clinics. Figure 1.1 identifies a number of learning facilitation roles, in an endeavour to distinguish the practice teacher role from these related roles.

Of course, these nursing and other healthcare profession learning facilitation titles need to be differentiated from a diverse range of titles in other health and social professions that comprise overlapping functions. Such titles include 'coach', which originates from sport, but has become a concept in its own right, as in 'life coaching' which tends to incorporate enabling physical fitness, exploring ways of achieving self-actualisation, and counselling. Rogers (2007: 176) suggests that the term coach refers to an individual who works with clients 'to achieve speedy, increased and sustainable effectiveness in their lives and careers through focused learning'. She indicates that the coach's sole aim is to guide the client to achieve his or her potential as defined by the client. The definition overlaps with education facilitation roles in healthcare, but can also be differentiated from them in that it directly addresses the whole person, and involves actions for personal change.

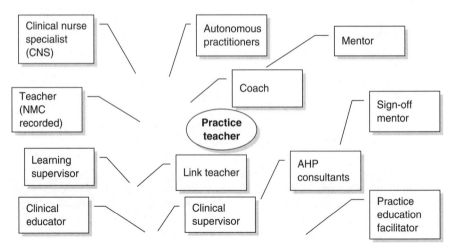

Figure 1.1   *Practice teacher and related learning support roles*

In addition to the practice-setting-based practice teacher, mentor, learning supervisor and other roles mentioned above for supporting learning and the assessment of competence in practice, other roles include personal tutor, PEF, lecturer-practitioners and link teachers. Depending on their job descriptions there is some overlap between these roles, but there are distinctions as well.

Brown (2006) explored the experiences of lecturer-practitioners in clinical practice for instance, and found that they tend to be in a position to work in partnership with practitioners to influence change and practice development in the clinical setting, as well as support continuing learning. Barrett (2007) explored developments in the clinical role of nurse lecturers, and concluded that this has been an ongoing debate that still needs resolving.

McArthur and Burns's (2008) report on an evaluation of PEF roles revealed that the role was welcomed by all groups of staff, although clinicians felt that PEFs should work mainly with students while PEFs themselves saw the main thrust of their roles as supporting mentors. Jowett and McMullan (2007) explored learning in practice through PEF roles, and found that PEFs are seen as supportive to both mentors and students and provide a vital link between the university and practice settings. The NMC (2009a) identifies a number of issues that PEFs address, such as the adequacy of resources to support the mentor role, and a lack of support for mentors when dealing with failing students and students with poor attitudes.

In an earlier study Brennan and Hutt (2001) examined the challenges and conflicts of facilitating learning in practice, and found that the role is problematic in various ways, as was the previous clinical teacher role. Clinical teaching in community nursing used to be provided by CPTs. Canham and Bennett (2002) argue that the healthcare professional with the relevant training for the CPT or equivalent role is crucial for supporting practice-based learning in all specialist areas of community practice, such as district nursing, health visiting, school nursing, community children's health nursing, community mental health nursing, community learning disabilities nursing, general practice nursing and occupational health nursing. Earlier on, Canham (1998) researched the educational support requirements of student specialist community practitioners, in particular in light of the then likely demise of the CPT role, and identified the valuable learning support contribution that CPTs made during practice placements, and therefore the need for this role. She recommended the provision of structured clinical supervision for novice CPTs.

However, there is already a 'critical mass' of experienced mentors who are fulfilling the practice teacher role in professional practice, and assessing students on specialist and advanced practice courses. In addition to several nursing roles with a relatively similar level of specialist responsibility, there is another layer of specialist roles in professions allied to medicine, for example consultant occupational therapist, senior dietician and medical registrar.

Akin to the practice teacher role in nursing, in social work, the term practice teacher increasingly refers to social care professionals who support learning for students on both pre- and post-qualifying social work courses (Walker et al., 2008), which coincides with efforts to galvanise social care with healthcare into a seamless service (e.g. DH, 2001a).

The developmental framework and practice teacher competences

The NMC (2008a) clearly identifies the specific criteria (Box 1.1) and competences of practice teachers for supporting learning and assessment in practice. The practice teacher role is seen as part of the developmental framework for supporting learning and assessment – see Figure 1.2, which suggests that all nurses and midwives have a duty to teach others, that at some point they will gain a mentor qualification, and possibly later in their career a practice teacher qualification, and subsequently an NMC teacher qualification that is required for nurse lecturers and PEF roles.

Competence and specific outcomes for each of the four stages of learning-support roles are identified under eight domains (top part of Figure 1.2), and the framework is also underpinned by five principles (A to E), which include being registered on the same part of the register as the student that the healthcare professional is supporting, holding appropriate level qualifications, and engagement in CPD.

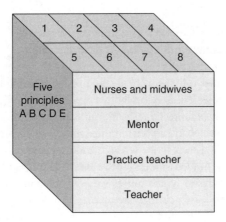

Figure 1.2   *The NMC's developmental framework*
Source: (NMC, 2008a)

It is mandatory for all SCPHN students to have a named qualified practice teacher for supporting learning and assessing nurses during their practice placement, and for students on SPQ and ANP courses. Qualified practice teachers may be part of the support for learning and assessment where this is a local requirement.

The NMC (2008a) identifies the outcomes that practice teachers must have developed on completion of an NMC approved practice teacher preparation programme, which will be cited when each domain is discussed in detail in subsequent chapters in this book. In addition to the criteria for practice teachers (Box 1.2), the NMC adds that qualified practice teachers are also responsible and accountable for:

- Organising and co-ordinating learning activities, primarily in practice learning environments for pre-registration students, and those intending to register as a SCPHN and SPQs where this is a local requirement.
- Supervising students and providing them with constructive feedback on their achievements.
- Setting and monitoring the achievement of realistic learning objectives in practice.
- Assessing total performance – including skills, attitudes and behaviours.
- Providing evidence as required by programme providers of a student's achievement or lack of achievement.
- Liaising with others (e.g. mentors, sign-off mentors, supervisors, personal tutors, the programme leader, other professionals) to provide feedback and identify any concerns about the student's performance and agree action as appropriate.
- Signing-off an achievement of proficiency at the end of the final period of practice learning or a period of supervised practice.

Practice teachers need allocated time for undertaking work with both pre-registration students, and with students on specialist or advanced practice programmes to enable them to facilitate students' learning and to assess the performance of relevant clinical skills. They normally work on a one-to-one basis with their student and use their professional judgement (e.g. Dowie and Elstein, 1988) and local/national policy to determine which activities may be safely delegated to students, as well as the level of supervision each one requires.

Factors driving specialist and advanced practice roles

Thus the practice teacher role incorporates supporting learning for students on SPQ and ANP programmes, as required locally by commissioners of healthcare-education programmes. Although definite policies and guidance are still awaited for specialist and advanced practice roles and associated titles, much has already been documented on how they are fulfilled in practice settings, and how they impact on patient care. For example, a jointly funded survey by the RCN (2005) and the Department of Health explored the ways in which nurses were working in advanced and extended roles, and also the ways in which they are proactive in developing roles and services. The survey findings highlighted the extensive range of services that contribute positively to service delivery and the quality of patient care, and the further potential for nurses carrying out these roles. However, it also revealed that time and funding constraints were holding some nurses back.

Why there are specialist and advanced practice roles

There are various factors that have instigated the proliferation of specialist and advanced practice roles, and evidence of the effectiveness in terms of patient outcomes is available. Included in Figure 1.1 are other roles that are equivalent to, or require a similar high level of, professional expertise as specialist and advanced nurse practitioners. Other current specialist and advanced practice roles include ANP, SCPHN, community matron, diabetes specialist nurse, modern matron, nurse consultant, nurse practitioner and outreach nurse.

These job titles emerged from significant changes in the way that services were delivered to patients by nurses undertaking treatment and care, which were previously in the domain of other healthcare professionals, notably doctors.

Action point 1.2 – Reasons for specialist and advanced practitioner roles

Drawing on your experience of specialist and advanced practice that you have observed or engaged with, make notes on (1) the various specific titles for several specialist and advanced-practitioner roles that you have encountered, or read about; and then on (2) why these specific specialist and advanced practice roles have been generated over recent years.

Callaghan (2008: 205) notes that there is a growing 'body of evidence indicating that advanced nursing practice results in an improvement in patient outcomes'. The development of specialist and advanced practice roles is triggered by local demand for specific healthcare services, which are often supported by government policies, which lead to nurses self-upskilling to provide for the local healthcare needs, and subsequently becoming specialists, or engaging in entrepreneurial activities in those areas. The more prominent driving policies and guidance that indicate the need for and the nature of specialist and advanced practice roles include the following.

- *Towards a Framework for Post-registration Nursing Careers – consultation response report* (DH, 2008a) and *Modernising Nursing Careers* (DH, 2006a) identify career pathways for nurses from the point of being a lay person and aspiring healthcare professional, to the point when they can become advanced practitioners.
- *High Quality Care for All – NHS Next Stage Review Final Report* (Darzi Report) (DH, 2008b) identifies eight clinical pathways for meeting local populations' healthcare needs by healthcare professionals, which can also comprise career pathways, the clinical pathways being: staying healthy (preventive service), maternity and newborn care, children's health, acute care, planned care, mental health, long-term conditions and end of life care.
- *RCN Competencies: Advanced nurse practitioners – an RCN guide to advanced nurse practitioner role, competencies and programme accreditation* (Royal College of Nursing [RCN], 2008) – as the title suggests, this document identifies the roles and competencies of ANPs.

- *A Reference Guide for Postgraduate Specialty Training in the UK* (Modernising Medical Careers [MMC], 2009) explains the career pathways and ways in which doctors can specialise after qualifying as a doctor and then successfully completing a two-year foundation programme.
- The NMC's position, as the professional regulator of nurses and midwives, in seeking to record SPQ and ANP qualifications on its professional register (NMC, 2008b).
- *Key Elements of the Career Framework*, as defined by the Skills for Health (2009a), wherein, for awards and qualifications, advanced practice is identified at Level 7 (of 9) – see Box 1.2.
- The *NHS Knowledge and Skills Framework* (DH, 2004a) identifies career pathways for healthcare staff, from being a lay person to becoming a very senior health-care professional, through the acquisition of knowledge and competence in core and specific dimensions at various levels of learning.
- *European Working Time Directive* (EWTD) (DH, 2009a) is the policy on a staged reduction of junior doctors' working hours, which have been reduced to 48 hours a week from August 2009.
- The Department of Health's Chief Nursing Officer's ten key roles for nurses iden-tified in *The NHS Plan* (DH, 2000) that nurses, midwives and therapists can develop their expertise in to provide prompter clinical services (see Box 1.3).
- *Care Closer to Home* (DH, 2008c) is a continuing project that has been set up to consider how care can be shifted and delivered in innovative ways to make it more locally accessible for patients and service users.

Box 1.2   Key elements of the career framework

More Senior Staff – Level 9
Staff with the ultimate responsibility for clinical caseload decision making and full on-call accountability.

Consultant Practitioners – Level 8
Staff working at a very high level of clinical expertise and/or have responsibility for the planning of services.

Advanced Practitioners – Level 7
Experienced clinical professionals who have developed their skills and theoret-ical knowledge to a very high standard. They are empowered to make high-level clinical decisions and will often have their own caseload. Non-clinical staff at Level 7 will typically be managing a number of service areas.

Senior Practitioners/Specialist Practitioners – Level 6
Staff who would have a higher degree of autonomy and responsibility than 'Practitioners' in the clinical environment, or who would be managing one or more service areas in the non-clinical environment.

Practitioners – Level 5
Most frequently registered practitioners in their first and second post-registration/ professional qualification jobs.

Assistant Practitioners/Associate Practitioners – Level 4
Probably studying for foundation degree, BTEC higher or HND. Some of their remit will involve them in delivering protocol-based clinical care that had previously been in the remit of registered professionals, under the direction and supervision of a state-registered practitioner.

Senior Healthcare Assistants/Technicians – Level 3
Have a higher level of responsibility than support worker, probably studying for, or having attained, an NVQ level 3 or Assessment of Prior Experiential Learning (APEL).

Support Workers – Level 2
Frequently with the job title of 'Healthcare Assistant' or 'Healthcare Technician' – probably studying for or have attained NVQ Level 2.

Initial Entry Level Jobs – Level 1
Such as 'Domestics' or 'Cadets' requiring very little formal education or previous knowledge, skills or experience in delivering or supporting the delivery of healthcare.

Source: Skills for Health, 2009a

Box 1.3   Chief Nursing Officer's ten key roles for nurses

- To order diagnostic investigations such as pathology tests and X-rays
- To make and receive referrals direct, say, to a therapist or a pain consultant
- To admit and discharge patients for specified conditions and within agreed protocols
- To manage patient caseloads, say for diabetes or rheumatology
- To run clinics, say, for ophthalmology or dermatology
- To prescribe medicines and treatments
- To carry out a wide range of resuscitation procedures including defibrillation
- To perform minor surgery and outpatient procedures
- To triage patients using the latest IT to the most appropriate health professional
- To take a lead in the way local health services are organised and in the way that they are run.

Source: DH, 2000

Healthcare professionals' career framework

The career framework for nurses and other healthcare professionals is predominantly initiated by national consultation documents and policies, and continues to evolve. Box 1.2 details the career framework for healthcare professionals as currently perceived by Skills for Health (2009a).

The implementation of standards for advanced nursing practice (e.g. NMC 2006a; RCN, 2008) is also dependent upon the outcomes of deliberations on the government White Paper on the regulation of healthcare professions, *Trust, Assurance and Safety – The Regulation of Health Professionals in the 21st Century* (DH, 2007a). It will also be influenced by the 'dimensions' of NHS posts identified in the *NHS KSF,* which the NMC (2006a) has mapped against advanced practice competencies; by the framework for post-registration qualifications when it is established by the four UK government health departments, as outlined by the DH (2006a); and the roles of specialist nurses with regard to the implementation of relevant National Service Frameworks (e.g. DH, 2001b).

Other key guidance publications include the MMC's (2009) post-qualifying career pathways for doctors. The DH (2008a) outlines the career pathways for nurses in five pathways, namely in: (1) children, family and public health, (2) first contact, access and urgent care, (3) supporting long-term care, (4) acute and critical care, and (5) mental-health and psychosocial care, which are based on patient pathways from newly qualified nurses to advanced practitioners with corresponding levels of education. These pathways guide and influence the content of both pre-registration nurse education and post-qualifying education programmes for nurses.

Contemporary nature of specialist and advanced practice

Since a wide variety of specialist and advanced practice roles, and posts have been developed over recent times, it is naturally moot to examine if there is a common thread across all specialist roles and across all advanced practice roles. This section now explores the exact nature of current specialist and advanced practice roles, and endeavours to ascertain healthcare professionals' and organisations' definitions and parameters of these roles.

What is specialist and advanced clinical practice?

As intimated above there are a number of perspectives on specialist and advanced practice roles, which are presented by relevant authorities such as the RCN, the International Council of Nurses (ICN), the DH, the NMC, and by research into the nature of these roles, and on the impact of these roles on patients' or service users' health and wellbeing. The Skills for Health's (2009a) nine levels of healthcare practitioners comprise one model of how these roles can be differentiated and developed during one's career (see Box 1.2).

Benner (2001) notes that skills are generally learnt and mastered over a span of time, on a continuum which starts from being a novice in the skill, to eventually becoming an expert. The continuum is as follows:

Novice ⟶ Advanced beginner ⟶ Competent ⟶ Proficient ⟶ Expert

Benner notes that becoming proficient, and eventually an expert, in specific clinical fields requires an extensive period of practice and experience, and ultimately expert practice in the level of practice that advanced healthcare professionals exercise. Nursing expertise is defined by Manley et al. (2005: 25) as 'the professional artistry and practice wisdom inherent in professional practice'. They add that the expert's professional artistry involves a blend of practitioner qualities, practice skills and creative-imagination processes. Concluding from a project that explored the nature of nursing expertise, they conclude that nursing expertise is prevalent in different roles, especially in those of CNSs, ANPs and consultant nurses.

CNSs are usually expert nurses for a specific client group, but ANPs' expertise is informed by skills in different disciplines, and their characteristics transcend clinical specialisms which can enable the seamless service associated with patient journeys. Manley (2008) describes nursing expertise as refined and integrated skills to a high level, which is nurtured and developed through not just on the length of time of practice, but also on predisposition, and the opportunities and support available.

Conway (1996) previously identified four types of experts, the first three of which she referred to as technologists, traditionalist and specialists who are all pragmatists, task orientated and medically dominated with little time for reflection, and the fourth type referred to as humanistic existentialists who rely on reflective practice to acquire their expertise.

The nature of specialist and advanced practice roles

The ICN (2001) recognises that advanced practice and CNS roles have been developing globally during the last two decades. Its definition of a nurse practitioner/ advanced practice nurse is: 'A registered nurse who has acquired the expert knowledge base, complex decision-making skills and clinical competencies for expanded practice, the characteristics of which are shaped by the context and/or country in which she is credentialed to practice' (p. 1).

The NMC's (2005b) consultation report on post-registration education shows that 70 per cent of respondents indicated that they preferred the title advanced nurse practitioner, 23 per cent the specialist nurse practitioner, while others suggested other titles. Many respondents commented that they preferred 'advanced' over 'specialist' as it better reflected higher-level practice, whilst specialist refers to the degree of specialisation within a particular field of practice, or sub-speciality.

The Association of Advanced Nursing Practice Educators (AANPE) (2009) is a UK organisation that supports specialist and advanced practitioners and plans relevant educational programmes. The AANPE indicates that it serves as a forum for various activities, including:

- Collaborative curriculum development and standard setting for ANP education across the four countries of the UK.
- Establishing the role and status of ANPs through an interface with other professions, professional and statutory bodies, commissioners, employers and relevant government bodies

Diverse specialist practice roles

Specialisation is prevalent in most healthcare and social-care professions. Doctors specialise, as do physiotherapists, occupational therapists and social workers, for instance. The Department of Health's (2001c) 'Advanced Letter' details the nature and requirements for nurse, midwife and allied health professions, consultant posts.

However, other than in medicine, registration of these senior level specialist posts on the profession's regulatory body's register is not standard practice at the moment.

In deciphering the areas of overlap and differences between specialist and ANP roles in different healthcare and social-care professions, it seems that there are also differences in the way nurses provide specialist and advanced practice care and treatment from the ways in which doctors do. Nurses take time and a more holistic approach to care and treatment, that is always taking into account the psychological, social, spiritual and cultural as well as physical factors that affect the individual's health. Generally nurses' salaries are also lower than those of doctors, which might comprise a more efficient use of health services' finances.

A number of instances of specific specialist and advanced practice activities that benefit patients and service users are discussed in Chapter 4 under practice development, as well as under evidence-based practice. As for SCPHNs, they work with both individuals and communities. In addition to their regular duties as nurses, they deal with issues related to the local population's health, and with new policies. The SCPHN Committee (NMC, 2009b: 1) defines the work of the SCPHN as follows:

> Specialist community public health nursing aims to reduce health inequalities by working with individuals, families, and communities promoting health, preventing ill health and in the protection of health. The emphasis is on partnership working that cuts across disciplinary, professional and organisational boundaries that impact on organised social and political policy to influence the determinants of health and promote the health of whole populations.

Educational preparation for the role is of one academic year's duration and awards a first degree and a NMC registerable qualification. However, there are ongoing issues related to SCPHNs in that there are too few health visitors, for instance, and also there is a lack of consensus about their role (McLellan, 2009).

Specialist and advanced practice roles and their specifications are still evolving, as healthcare trusts develop these roles to meet local patients' and service users' care and treatment needs in the form of local specialist services. It often requires nurses' upskilling into unprecedented roles, and in some of the roles previously occupied by doctors, for example non-medical prescribing. A case study based on an innovation cited in *Our Health, Our Care, Our Say: Making It Happen* (DH, 2006b) in relation to 'care closer to home' illustrates this.

Case study: Better services for people with long-term conditions in Dudley

In Rose-hill PCT the development of new roles has risen markedly, such as the 'Community Heart Failure Service' that involves nurses conducting community clinics and providing a home-treatment service to prevent patients having to travel to hospital. The nurse takes a holistic view of the patient, which includes assessing wider environmental factors alongside clinical symptoms. Strong links remain with hospital consultants, so that specialist opinions can be obtained very quickly. With the growing expertise of these nurses and the fact that some members of the team can now prescribe many of the drugs necessary for fast, effective treatment this means that a deterioration in the patient's condition can be prevented very quickly. Patients feel that the home-treatment service helps them to stay safely at home with their family rather than having to attend the hospital.

A number of research studies have been conducted on the impact of CNSs' roles. Maughan and Clarke (2001), for instance, report on a randomised controlled trial (RCT) that found that sexual functioning and quality of life were improved in the group that received specialist psychosexual counselling following treatment for gynaecological cancer. However, a RCN survey (Mooney, 2008a) report on CNSs reveals that only half of all CNSs feel that the work they do are valued by their trusts, and more than 30 per cent feel that they are at risk of redundancy. This is despite research findings that CNSs' work is more cost-effective than that of doctors.

The clinical activities of CNSs are also captured by a computer program named 'Pandora' that comprises a record of all clinical activities that CNSs perform, and their outcomes (Waters, 2007). These activities are grouped under eight dimensions, and when three days of activities are inputted, the program can generate histograms and pie charts to demonstrate the impact of particular CNSs on patient outcomes. It is claimed that the program also captures the non-hands-on care activities that CNSs engage in such as preventive unscheduled care. The implications of this program are discussed further in Chapter 8.

Advanced nurse practitioners

In *The Proposed Framework for the Standard for Post-Registration Nursing*, the NMC (2008b: 1) defines advanced-nurse practitioners as '... highly experienced and educated members of the care team who are able to diagnose and treat your health care needs or refer you to an appropriate specialist if needed'. They expand on the definition and specify that ANPs are highly skilled nurses who can:

- take a comprehensive patient history;
- carry out physical examinations;
- use their expert knowledge and clinical judgement to identify the potential diagnosis;
- refer patients for investigations where appropriate;
- make a final diagnosis;
- decide on and carry out treatment, including the prescribing of medicines, or refer patients to an appropriate specialist;
- use their extensive practice experience to plan and provide skilled and competent care to meet patients' healthcare and social-care needs, involving other members of the healthcare team as appropriate;
- ensure the provision of continuity of care including follow-up visits;
- assess and evaluate, with patients, the effectiveness of the treatment and care provided and make changes as needed;
- work independently, although often as part of a healthcare team;
- provide leadership; and
- ensure that each patient's treatment and care are based on best practice.

The NHS Scotland (Scottish Government, 2008) drew the key elements from several definitions of specialist and advanced practice roles together with the aim of facilitating a common understanding and guiding the further development of these roles, including those cited above, and it proposes its own definition of advanced nursing practice as:

- Advanced practice is a 'level of practice' rather than a role or title.
- The career framework for health articulates 'advanced practitioners' across professional boundaries.
- Advanced practice is shown across four key themes:
  o advanced clinical/professional practice
  o facilitating learning
  o leadership/management
  o research.

- These themes are underpinned by autonomous practice, critical thinking, high levels of decision making and problem solving, values-based care and improving practice.
- The skills and knowledge base for advanced practice are influenced by the context in which individuals practise.

The RCN (2008) also provides its own definition of ANP along similar lines with a number of bullet points, and states that educational preparation for the role must at minimum be first degree honours level.

Skills for Health (2009a: 1) defines Advanced Practitioners (level 7) as: 'Experienced clinical professionals who have developed their skills and theoretical knowledge to a very high standard. They are empowered to make high-level clinical decisions and will often have their own caseload. Non-clinical staff at Level 7 will typically be managing a number of service areas' – as noted in Box 1.3. It also identifies a number of specific competencies for each level for the different healthcare professions.

On the other hand, the NMC (2008c) suggests that there are nurses who hold job titles that imply an advanced level of knowledge and competence, but who do not actually possess such knowledge and competence. Furthermore, their practice may not be subject to scrutiny by another professional as they will often act as independent practitioners.

The NMC indicates that the ANP qualification should be recorded on the NMC's professional register, and it is seeking approval from the Privy Council for doing so. However, the NMC needs to identify a mechanism for monitoring how practitioners demonstrate their continued fitness for practice after having their qualifications recorded on the NMC register. It recognises that the advanced-practice debate will also have to address the relationship of ANP qualifications to other parts of the register, should a 'fitness to practice' issue arise around a lack of competence.

Successful achievement of specialist and advanced practice standards of proficiency currently leads to qualifications being recorded on the nurses' part of the register for specialist practice in the fields of adult, mental health, learning disabilities or children's nursing, and the specialist community qualifications of district nursing, general practice nursing, community child nursing, community learning disabilities nursing and community mental health nursing as identified in Box 1.5 later in this chapter. The NMC indicates that only nurses who have achieved the NMC's competencies for registered ANPs are permitted to use the title, which will therefore be protected through a registerable qualification in the NMC's register.

The competencies in which the ANP will have to demonstrate capability and expertise in order to be able to have their qualification recorded on the NMC register are identified in the learning beyond initial registration document (NMC, 2005b). They are identified under seven domains, which are very similar to those identified by the RCN (2008), both building on preceding work on the subject area – see Box 1.4.

Box 1.4   Areas of expertise for ANPs

	NMC (2005b) domains for learning beyond initial registration	*RCN (2008) domains for Advanced Nurse Practitioners*
Domain 1:	The nurse–patient relationship	Assessment and management of patient health/illness status
Domain 2:	Respecting culture and diversity	The nurse–patient relationship
Domain 3:	Management of patient health/ illness status	The education function
Domain 4:	The education function	Professional role
Domain 5:	Professional role	Managing and negotiating healthcare delivery systems
Domain 6:	Managing and negotiating healthcare delivery systems	Monitoring and ensuring the quality of advanced healthcare practice
Domain 7:	Monitoring and ensuring the quality of healthcare practice	Respecting culture and diversity

However, the decision to record ANP qualifications on the NMC's professional register suggests that this is a role beyond specialisation. Advanced practice is a career progression point when the healthcare professional has moved beyond generalist/generic clinical skills, and has gained specialist skills to a level of expertise that utilises broader problem-solving and critical thinking skills.

Research on the ANP role includes a study by Gardner et al. (2007) which concludes with the 'Strong Model of Advanced Practice' as an operational framework for the implementation and evaluation of these roles, with competencies under the headings:

- Direct comprehensive care.
- Support of systems.
- Education.
- Research.
- Publication and professional leadership.

An English National Board for Nursing, Midwifery and Health Visiting (ENB) sponsored study that evaluated the outcomes of an advanced neonatal nurse practitioner programme concluded that the role of advanced neonatal nurses was valued (Renshaw et al., 1999), but educational preparation programmes for this role were diverse across educational institutions, and standardisation was needed for a more universal definition of this role. The clinical conditions requiring specialist and advanced practice interventions are related to emergency care, long-term conditions, and so on, educational preparation for which leads to university awards as are identified shortly in this chapter.

Modern matrons and consultant nurses

Modern matrons and community matrons are other recent specialist roles developed for nurses with appropriate expertise in several areas, such as acute hospital wards, in mental health and in primary care. Clegg and Bee (2008) report on the findings of a survey of patients' and carers' views about a new community matron service, for instance, the strengths of which include the reliability of the service, the confidence it gave to patients and carers, the improved links with GP services and the likelihood of preventing admission to hospital. They recommend continued investment in the community matron service.

Beyond specialist and advanced practice roles are nurse consultant posts that emerged from research (e.g. Manley, 2000), and were then implemented through the Department of Health (2001c) directive. Nurse-consultant posts in many specialisms have been documented (e.g. Manley, 2000; Burton et al., 2009). More recent research on nurse consultants (e.g. Coster et al., 2006; Redwood et al., 2007) tends to indicate that they have a positive impact in improving the service provided to the clientele group, as well as in leadership and consultancy, education and training, practice development and research.

Healthcare consultant roles feature prominently in the Darzi report (DH, 2008b). It recommends the creation of community specialist consultant posts for healthcare professionals in order to see patients in GP surgeries and primary care centres to treat long-term conditions such as diabetes and heart disease earlier and faster, and thus prevent complications.

Educational preparation for specialist and advanced practice

Naturally, the effective fulfilment of CNS and ANP roles requires the relevant educational preparation. Until around 2002, specialist nurses were relatively easy to recognise in that they had a post-registration specialist qualification that had been approved by the ENB (1991) as part of a framework for continuing professional education for nurses and midwives, and the ENB issued certificates for these qualifications, and also held a record of nurses and midwives with specialist qualifications.

Since the ENB was dismantled following a management consultancy report that highlighted weaknesses in the way they operated, these records are no longer held centrally. Subsequently, when the NMC replaced the UKCC, whose policies were operationalised by the four national Boards in the UK, the recording of specialist and advanced practice qualifications has been dysfunctional. The post-qualifying qualifications that are recorded on the NMC register are cited in Box 1.5.

Box 1.5   Recorded/registered specialist qualifications

Code	Specialist qualification
RHV	Specialist Community Public Health Nursing – HV (Health visiting)
RSN	Specialist Community Public Health Nursing – SN (School nursing)
ROH	Specialist Community Public Health Nursing – OH (Occupational health)
RFHN	Specialist Community Public Health Nursing – FHN (Family Health Nurse)
V100	Mode 1 Prescribing
V200	Extended Nurse Prescribing
V300	Extended/Supplementary Nursing Prescribing
TCH	Teacher
SPAN	Specialist Practitioner – Adult Nursing
SPMH	Specialist Practitioner – Mental Health
SPCN	Specialist Practitioner – Children's Nursing
SPLD	Specialist Practitioner – Learning Disability Nurse
SPGP	Specialist Practitioner – General Practice Nursing
SCMH	Specialist Practitioner – Community Mental Health Nursing
SCLD	Specialist Practitioner – Community Learning Disabilities Nursing
SPCC	Specialist Practitioner – Community Children's Nursing
SPDN	Specialist Practitioner – District Nursing

Source: NMC, 2009c

Nonetheless, education programmes in healthcare specialisms have to continue, in order to meet service needs, and currently universities offer specialist courses either as multiple modules, or as a first or Master's degree-awarding programme. The specialist or advanced practice qualification appears in the student's transcript, usually together with details of the modules that were successfully completed by the student as the 120-credit-point final year of a degree programme, which are focused on the clinical skills and knowledge required for the specialist or advanced practice role. The 120-point course is likely to incorporate modules on research and leadership as they are considered essential for those holding specialist and advanced practitioner posts. At post-graduate level, for each specialist and advanced practice subject area, the qualifications generally awarded are:

- a post-graduate certificate (60 credit points at level 7)
- a post-graduate diploma (120 credit points at level 7)
- a Master's degree (180 credit points at level 7).

For example, the specialist areas for registered children's nurses include neonatal nursing, community children's nursing and teenagers and young adults with cancer. They are normally studied at post-graduate certificate, post-graduate diploma or Master's degree level, although programmes at a first degree level also continue to be offered. The programmes that are recorded on the NMC register require NMC approval. Awards for these specialist and advanced practice programmes include a Post-Graduate Certificate in:

- acute and critical care
- advanced skills in neonatal practice
- end of life care
- long-term conditions, e.g. diabetes
- mental health
- paediatric cardiothoracic care
- public health
- teenagers and young adults with cancer.

Research on the educational preparation for specialist or advanced practitioners includes a study by Girot and Rickaby (2008) who evaluated the educational preparation of community matrons who work with patients with complex long-term conditions, and can meet the specifications of *Modernising Nursing Careers* (DH, 2006a). They used a mixed methods approach to data collection, including documentary analysis, self-administered questionnaires, individual telephone interviews and focus groups undertaken with the education programme development team. The study revealed that the majority of students believed that the programme had met their expectations and had helped them to fulfil the functions of the community matron role as defined in national competence statements. However, a number of respondents indicated that they experienced difficulties with the level of organisational support available, such as lack of facilitation for their work-based learning, and therefore Girot and Rickaby highlight a need for organisations to develop their infrastructure to support new roles as well as offer protected time for learning in practice.

Educational preparation for practice teacher role

The NMC's (2008a) guidance and requirements for educational preparation programmes for practice teachers are as follows:

- Include at least 30 days' protected learning time – to include learning in both academic and practice settings.
- Include relevant work-based learning with the opportunity to reflect critically on such an experience, e.g. acting as a practice teacher to a student in specialist practice under the supervision of a qualified practice teacher.
- Meet the additional criteria for a sign-off mentor.
- Should normally be completed within six months.
- The content of a previous mentor programme, where appropriate, may be accredited, enabling the practice teacher programme to be completed in less time.

Practice teacher programmes are developed in response to the need for practice teachers in local healthcare trusts, and they build on healthcare professionals' existing expertise in mentoring. They are normally at post-graduate level and delivered over a 26-week period, and should include at least 30 days' protected learning time in academic and practice settings. The latter constitute work-based learning, where students are supported by an overall learning supervisor, who provides the practice teacher student the opportunity to reflect critically on practice experiences. The teaching and learning strategy includes meeting the additional criteria for a sign-off mentor (as indicated by the NMC, 2008a), and provides a foundation for undertaking an NMC-approved teacher preparation programme. The course can be offered as a core or an optional component of an MSc advanced nursing practice programme, for instance, or as a more generic MSc in Health Studies.

Practice teacher courses recognise the practice teacher's responsibility in enabling students to achieve specialist or advanced healthcare competencies, and in assessing them to ascertain fitness to practise. Courses therefore address the knowledge and competence necessary to fulfil the practice teacher role, and on completion of the preparation programme qualified practice teachers are responsible and accountable for their teaching and assessing roles and for making decisions in relation to the competence of students on specialist or advanced practice programmes. During the course they are supported and assessed by a practice-based learning supervisor with the appropriate educational qualifications and motivation, and they also need to have access to pre-registration students who are at the sign-off proficiency stage of their course, and to post-qualifying students on specialist or advanced practice courses.

On successful completion of the NMC-approved practice teacher preparation programme, registrants taking the practice teacher role should have developed competence and been assessed by their learning supervisor on the achievement of all 26 outcomes for a practice teacher. They will also have developed such cognitive (thinking) skills as (NMC, 2008a):

- Evaluating research and a variety of types of information and evidence critically.
- Synthesising information from a number of sources in order to gain a coherent understanding of theory and practice.
- Analysing, evaluating and interpreting the evidence underpinning practice teaching and learning, and managing change in practice appropriately.
- Evaluating inter-professional learning in practice teaching and learning activities.
- Evaluating ways in which students develop specialist and advanced practice knowledge and competence.

Healthcare professionals who have previously successfully completed a similar programme (e.g. CPT) can use the healthcare trust's self-declaration form to indicate that they are up to date with their professional practice, as well as with the NMC's practice teacher outcomes, and then continue in the role of practice teacher. They can also use the university's AP(E)L mechanism to gain credit points towards a relevant university award.

Practice teacher students who successfully complete the course have their names recorded on the locally held register for mentors and practice teachers. They are thereafter required to update and develop their knowledge and competence, attend annual updates and undergo a triennial review, as required by the NMC (2008a).

Conclusion

Chapter 1 of this textbook began by exploring the rationales for the practice teacher role, the criteria that have to be met to hold the title legitimately and the scope of the role. The latter included distinguishing the practice teacher role from related roles such as mentor, NMC-approved teacher and learning supervisor. Subsequently, the factors driving specialist and advanced practice were explored, and included career pathways for healthcare professionals. The contemporary nature of specialist and advanced practice was also examined, including the current debates and research on inherent components of these concepts; and finally the educational preparation for specialist and advanced practitioners, and for the practice teacher role.

It therefore focused on:

- The nature of, and rationales for, the practice teaching role, including the NMC's (2008a) developmental framework; the criteria and scope of practice teaching; distinctions between the practice teacher and similar roles; and the practice teacher's role in facilitating learning and assessing the competence of students on specialist and advanced practice courses.
- An exploration of the factors driving specialist and advanced practice roles, and current developments leading to nurses' upskilling to provide a local needs-based health service, and subsequently becoming specialist in those areas; contemporary knowledge and evidence of the effectiveness of specialist and advanced practice roles in terms of patient outcomes; and modernising healthcare professionals' careers.
- Contemporary perspectives on specialist and advanced practice, including current definitions and characteristics, deliberations and reviews of competencies at levels beyond initial registration, and specialist practice and advanced nurse practitioners' qualifications; and the clinical contexts in which specialist and advanced practice are delivered.
- The educational preparation for specialist and advanced practice roles, and for the practice teacher role, taking into account the NMC's (2008a) practice teacher stan-dards as the criteria for supporting the learning and assessment of specialist and advanced practice competence.

The practice teacher role is pretty much well identified. As for specialist and advanced practitioner roles, whilst so far there have been suggestions over various aspects, it seems that a consensus is imminent, with the primary beneficiary being patients and service users. How the practice teacher establishes, manages and maintains working relationships with students, colleagues, patients or service users, and with the members of medical and other non-medical professions, is the focus of Chapter 2.

2

Establishing and Managing Effective Working Relationships as a Practice Teacher

Introduction

Having examined the rationales for the practice-teaching role and its scope, along with the competencies for CNSs and ANPs, and the current contexts in which specialist and advanced practitioners work, Chapter 2 focuses on how working interpersonal relationships are formed particularly between practice teachers and their students.

Chapter outcomes

On completion of this chapter you should be able to:

1. Identify a number of reasons for practice teachers needing to form, establish, maintain and manage interpersonal relationships with various healthcare professionals, and with students in their field of practice.
2. Evaluate ways in which psychosocial development influences the formation of effective working relationships between individuals in general.
3. Analyse the actions that practice teachers and students take to ensure that an effective professional relationship is established.
4. Evaluate ways of supporting pre-registration and post-qualifying students to enable them to acquire specialist or advanced practice knowledge and competence, and to achieve their practice placement objectives.
5. Explore the ways in which practice teachers form effective intra- and inter-professional relationships within an ethos of inter-professional learning.
6. Analyse potential problematic interpersonal relationship situations that might develop in practice teaching, and the actions that can be taken to avert or resolve them.

Reasons for developing and establishing working relationships

Healthcare professionals have to develop and establish effective working relationships with others, including students, patients or service users, the aim of which is to achieve the purpose of the relationship, which for students is to maximise learning during practice placements.

Why explore 'working' relationships?

A working relationship and understanding between the practice teacher and the student they are supervising is essential for the latter's learning to be effective. This comprises a rapport between them that is based on theories and principles of relationship building (e.g. Rogers and Freiberg, 1994; Crawford et al., 2000).

Concepts related to interpersonal relationships include a 'rapport' between two individuals, or the lack of it. Rapport has to be cultivated and established very early on in the practice teacher–student contact to ensure the aims of the placement are achieved in good time. It is also one of the NMC's (2004b) 'standards of proficiency' for all nurses and midwives, as well as a standard for practice teachers. Indeed, the NMC (2008a) indicates that the registered nurse who is competent as a practice teacher must be able to:

- Have effective professional and inter-professional working relationships to support learning for entry to the register, and education at a level beyond initial registration.
- Be able to support students moving into specific areas of practice – or a level of practice beyond initial registration, identifying their individual needs when moving to a different level of practice.
- Support mentors and other professionals in their role to support learning across practice and academic learning environments.

The above outcomes reflect the practice teacher's ability to form working relationships that are effective and ample to support learning for pre-registration students, for post-qualifying registrants, for newly qualified mentors, and other students on learning beyond initial registration programmes across practice and academic learning environments. It refers to the practice teacher's ability to demonstrate an understanding of those factors that influence how students integrate into clinical settings; to provide ongoing and constructive support to facilitate the transition from one learning environment to another; and to develop effective professional and inter-professional working relationships to support learning as part of a wider inter-professional team.

In common with nurse lecturers and mentors as facilitators of learning, practice teachers also have a pastoral role towards students. Webb and Shakespeare (2007) explored how mentors make judgements about students' clinical competence, and concluded that good learning support depends to a large extent on students themselves initiating and building a relationship with their mentors. They emphasise that in their view 'much of the burden of creating effective mentoring relationships falls on students' (p. 563). They also found that issues identified in previous research, such as a lack of time for mentoring and insufficient support for mentors, had still not been resolved. Similar issues could prevail with the practice teacher student relationship unless the practice teacher implements an informed strategy for ensuring effective working relationships with all their students are formed.

The nature and dynamics of interpersonal relationships

Price (2005) refers to the teacher–student relationship in clinical settings as a 'learning relationship', and suggests that there are four stages of building 'learning relationships', which are: (1) initially the teacher and mentee recognise that they are 'strangers' and start to communicate; (2) as 'explorers' they get to know the other as a person and ascertain ways of facilitating learning; (3) as 'companions' they get on with their respective roles as teacher and learner; and (4) as 'network associates', i.e. they still keep in touch after the placement ends.

Action point 2.1   How do you establish effective personal relationships?

Consider the more enduring relationships that you have experienced so far (as opposed to fleeting or casual encounters), and make notes on how you established each of these relationships, and how you sustained them, when you chose to.

Lifers

We develop different degrees of relationships with a wide range of people in our personal and professional lives. To begin to analyse how these relationships are built, it is important first to identify who we build relationships with. This comprises our 'role-set', which refers to a multiplicity of roles that are associated with, or attached to, a major role that an individual holds. An instance of this can be identified by jotting down on a sheet of paper all the people you interact with in a meaningful way in addition to those in your domestic life. The likely professional role-set for practice teachers is depicted in Figure 2.1, the components of which also comprise their responsibility or accountability. The relationships identified in the role-set diagram excludes casual encounters and acquaintances such as the postman, shop-keepers and so on, if encounters with them are limited to one or two very brief and fleeting exchanges.

An effective relationship in the work or clinical setting can be defined as one that comprises acceptance of each other by the two parties involved, establishing a mutual understanding and rapport, which might constitute small negotiations and giving time, and require intrapersonal awareness and interpersonal skills such as empathic listening. An effective professional relationship in healthcare requires fulfilling all components of this definition, as well as a full awareness of those components that each is responsible and accountable for. There must also be adherence to work related protocols and policies, and to professional codes of practice.

As social beings we all have enduring relationships at various points in our lives. This may be based on blood relationships such as with our kin, those relationships that develop in our social endeavours and encounters, at work, and those that we deliberately create for specific purposes.

Interpersonal communication

Communication is a fundamental requirement for developing effective interpersonal relationships. It is useful to distinguish between two levels of communication, foundation level and specialist level. Foundation-level communication comprises the verbal and non-verbal communication that we all normally acquire during

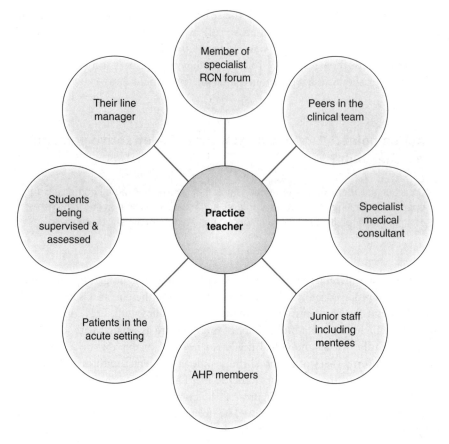

Figure 2.1   *Professional role-set requiring a working relationship – the practice teacher*

our developmental years, and use in day-to-day activities. Specialist level communications are those that require specialist training so that they can be used for specific purposes, usually professional. There are different modes of foundation level communication:

- Written verbal communication – i.e. by letter, email, printed material, faxed.
- Spoken verbal communication – using selected words from the language.
- Non-verbal aspects of spoken verbal communication – e.g. tone of voice, volume and emphasis – which can be face-to-face, over the telephone, video conferencing, etc.
- Non-verbal communication without spoken words (non-vocal) – e.g. gestures, degree of proximity, facial expression and body orientation.

Argyle (1994) suggests that there are various facets to non-verbal communication, such as:

- Non-verbal signals being more powerful for communicating emotions and inter-personal attitudes than verbal ones.
- Some aspects of communication are socially safer to present non-verbally – such as one's self-presentation and negative attitudes – than verbally.

Furthermore, non-verbal communication is utilised to supplement and reinforce verbal communication. Specialist level communication is usually utilised in specific formal encounters that are constituted for a particular purpose such as when being interviewed for a professional post, conducting a meeting and counselling.

Research on 'establishing working relationships' includes a study by Burnard and Morrison (1989) which revealed that some of the personal qualities of an interpersonally skilled or competent person include being approachable, empathic, helpful, genuine, a good listener, verbally skilled, an acceptor of self, open and credible. We develop the attributes of the interpersonally skilled or competent person over an extended period of time through our psychosocial development, as identified by Erikson (1995) for instance.

Psychosocial development

Interpersonal skills are developed through interpersonal interaction, and therefore referred to as psychosocial development. Erikson (1995) researched how individuals learn to build relationships during the course of their lifetime, and he consequently constituted his theory of 'Stages of psychosocial development'. Erikson suggested that we go through eight stages of development, each of which encompasses a time span of development when we encounter a particular form of 'psychosocial crisis' which, if successfully resolved, comprises learning and influences development in the next stage. These stages of psychosocial development in brief are as follows:

1   Infancy (birth–18 months): during this time span, which Erikson refers to as the 'trust vs mistrust' stage, the child develops trust in others around him, and to achieve this, he needs maximum comfort and minimal uncertainty in relating to others, and to the environment.
2   Toddler (1½–3 years): this is the stage when the child endeavours to master his physical environment by tentative exploration of items in the environment and endeavouring to communicate with others, thereby resolving the psychosocial crisis 'autonomy vs shame and doubt'.
3   Preschool or play age (3–6 years): 'initiative vs guilt' is the psychosocial crisis experienced by the pre-school child when they begin to initiate, not imitate, activities, and depending on the feedback gained from those around him, develops a conscience and sexual identity.
4   School-age child (7–10 years): 'industry vs inferiority' is experienced when the school-age child tries to develop a sense of self-worth by refining their skills.
5   Adolescence (10–17 years): during adolescence, the psychosocial crisis encountered by the individual is 'identity vs role confusion', and this is when the individual tries integrating many roles (child, sibling, student, athlete, worker) into a self-image, and is influenced by role models and peer pressure.
6   Young adulthood (18–40 years): the psychosocial crisis experienced in young adulthood is 'intimacy vs isolation', when the individual explores and learns to form a personal relationship and commitment to another as partner or spouse.
7   Middle adulthood (40–65 years): 'generativity vs stagnation' is experienced in middle adulthood when the individual seeks to gain satisfaction through productivity in career, family and civic interests.

8   Later adulthood (from 65 years): characterised by a time to review own life's accom-
    plishments, the psychosocial crisis experienced is '*integrity vs despair*,' and generally
    comprises retirement from full-time employment and a readiness for substantial spare
    time for the rest of own life.

Erikson (1995) therefore maintains that we develop psychosocially in a predetermined
order, which in turn affects our sense of self. Each of the above eight distinct stages
can result in two possible outcomes – a successful completion of the stages resulting
in a healthy personality based on successful interactions with others, or a failure to
complete a stage successfully can result in a reduced ability to complete further stages,
and therefore possibly a less healthy personality and perception of self. These crises,
however, can be resolved successfully later on in life.

The individuals who practice teachers supervise include pre-qualifying students
entering nursing as a career, and therefore can be anywhere between 18 years of
age to those in their mid-50s. From adulthood onwards, according to Erikson, the
individual experiences intimacy or isolation, generativity or stagnation, and
integrity versus despair in sequence. A successful resolution of these crises results
in an emotionally more mature and psychosocially more skilled individual, but
unsatisfactory outcomes are reflected in states of 'isolation', 'stagnation' or 'despair'.

For the more mature entrant, they may have had various life experiences, be
skilled in numerous social or vocational dimensions, and have their own learning
styles and expectations.

The practice teacher can therefore take into account their students' likely stages
of psychosocial development in terms of building working relationships, as positive
outcomes of these crises result in the individual's subsequent degree of ability
to build and sustain a more productive learning relationship with their practice
teacher. Negative outcomes might obstruct this process.

Yet another perspective with regard to the teacher–student relationship is that
of social development as represented in Bandura's (1977) social learning theory
which explores the dynamics of learning skills from a skilled individual. Social
learning theory is discussed in the context of learning clinical skills in Chapter 3.

Working relationships in healthcare

The nurse–patient relationship

The very widely adopted principles of building trusting and effective relationships
advocated by Rogers and Freiberg's (1994), which are also required for building a
'therapeutic relationship' in counselling and therapeutic communication scenarios,
comprise three key conditions:

- *Acceptance, trust*: accepting each person for who they are, what they look like, for
  their strengths and weaknesses, showing and feeling trust in each other.
- *Genuineness, respect*: being honest about one's knowledge and competence, and
  about areas that still need developing; showing mutual respect.
- *Empathic understanding*: being able to see eventualities from another person's
  standpoint.

Self-awareness and appropriate self-disclosure can be added to this list. Further-more, Burnard and Morrison (2005) explored nurses' self-perception of their interpersonal skills using Heron's (1989) six-category intervention analysis with a convenient sample of 93 qualified nurses, and found that nurses perceive themselves as more skilled in authoritative categories (prescriptive, informative, confronting), and less skilled in facilitative categories (cathartic, catalytic, supportive). The authors suggest that the findings have implications for curriculum design. Naturally it is useful if the practice teacher is skilled in the utilisation of these specialist interpersonal skills. Alternatively, if the situation requires, they can refer to agencies such as Occupational Health who should have knowledge of how to access personnel who have these skills, such as appointed counsellors.

Waters (2008) explored the qualities that patients rate in nurses, and found these to be: attentiveness, caring, organisation, professionalism, kindness, sympathy, cheerfulness, thoughtfulness, selflessness, advocacy, efficiency and politeness. These qualities would therefore comprise a precondition for forming nurse–patient relationships. May (1990) examined theoretical and educational literature on interpersonal relations between nurses and patients, and concluded that there are two contending perspectives. One is characterised by technocratic factors, which are task-oriented, routinised and superficial interactions by the nurse; and the other is contextual factors whereupon nurses engage in meaningful conversation with patients about their health, and therefore forming a more health-benefiting relationship for the patient.

Furthermore, Arnold and Boggs (2003) distinguish between levels of involve-ment between the two parties (which is the practice teacher–student relationship in the context of this book), which are (1) detached, (2) helpful, or (3) over-involved. Neither the first nor the third type of involvement is desirable if the student's placement objectives are to be achieved.

On exploring how mental health nurses develop effective interpersonal relations with service users, a skill that is of critical significance in mental-health nursing, Peplau (1987) concluded that this is a complex process that comprises three overlapping phases, from getting acquainted (orientation), to working and then eventually terminating the relationship. The working phase is when the majority of 'active intervention' is executed.

Ferari (2006) explored academic education's contribution to the development of nurse–patient relationships, and found that teaching methods such as reflection, seminars, role plays, case studies and group discussions enable students to develop a more efficacious relationship with their patients.

The student–teacher relationship in practice teaching

Crawford et al. (2000) explored final-year student nurses' experience of mentors (referred to as preceptors in the article) which indicated that the mentor–mentee relationship is 'pivotal' to student learning. The components that are essential for building this relationship include:

- *Creating a safe environment for learning* – i.e. arranging orientation activities, relevant observational experiences, and preventing or dealing with errors and miscon-ceptions, etc.

- *Teaching strategies employed by preceptors* – e.g. role-modelling, providing support and encouragement, and giving relevant information.
- *Soloing* – which refers to students who are deemed competent in relevant skills working independent of their mentor in care delivery.

These components are also applicable to the practice teacher–student relationship, and are largely consistent with Peplau's (1987) three-phase relationship formation, with the second phase comprising the student engaging in caring for service users independent of the practice teacher, albeit under their guidance and indirect supervision.

From another perspective, Wilkes (2006) reviewed the literature on the student–mentor relationship, and concluded that as this learning support role is performed as one of multiple roles, for the relationship to be effective and not compromised, mentors should exercise caution and set clear boundaries at the very outset. She suggests that both parties will then have realistic expectations of each other and reduce the likelihood of misunderstanding and mistrust. Furthermore, ground rules for the placement should be established at the initial interview and documented in the learning contract.

However, Agnew (2005) acknowledges that a good student–mentor relationship is not always easy to achieve, especially if individual healthcare professionals are reluctant to accept the mentoring role. These mentors are those that 'tick boxes' rather than teach and assess students, and consequently contribute to 'a vicious circle of incompetence' (p. 26).

How to develop effective working and learning relationships

Having ascertained the various factors that can influence the formation of effective relationships between individuals, and those between nurses and patients or service users, and between healthcare professionals and their students, the chapter now focuses on the strategies and approaches that practice teachers can adopt to facilitate effective working and learning relationships with both pre-registration students and qualified colleagues, which can also include the use of learning contracts or learning agreements.

Davies and Gilling (1998) make some very straightforward recommendations on how a learning facilitator can build relationships with students. They indicate that these involve preparing for the student's arrival, beginning the facilitator–student relationship and supporting the student during the practice placement, and include:

- Preparing for and arranging the first meeting with the student at the very beginning of the placement, ensuring that they are given full attention.
- Welcoming the student with enthusiasm and interest.
- Orientating the student to the clinical environment.
- Finding out about the student's past experiences.
- Clarifying mutual expectations.
- Setting ground rules.

Levett-Jones et al. (2009) explored whether pre-registration students' feeling of belongingness to the clinical team during practice placements had any effect on students' learning experiences, and found that it is an essential ingredient for both learning and a positive clinical experience. They suggested that receptiveness, inclusion, a legitimisation of the student role, recognition, challenge and support had the most important influence on students' sense of belonging and learning. Levett-Jones et al. also suggested that nursing students' motivation and capacity to learn, self-concept, confidence, the extent to which they were willing to question or conform to poor practice, and their future career decisions are influenced by the extent to which they experience belongingness to the team.

Effective practice teaching by role modelling

The characteristics of effective mentors have been identified though research (e.g. Kelly, 2007). Those of a good nurse have also been variously explored, and Waters' (2008) findings were identified earlier in this chapter. However, documentation of the specific characteristics of a good or effective practice teacher is scarce because it is still a very novel role. Nonetheless, the same principles that underpin building a teacher–student relationship in other learning facilitation roles should apply to the practice teacher role as well.

One of the characteristics that is increasingly being highlighted is that all nurses need to be role models, and that this should not be limited to the work environment, but included in their personal comportment as well, in particular in relation to leading healthier lifestyles (e.g. *Nursing Standard News*, 2008a).

In general, a model is a simplified representation of a complex concept. The nurse as a role model could be represented by a set of attributes. Coady (2003), for instance, summarising the attributes of consultant nurses, indicates that they constitute being role models in four areas:

- Expert practice.
- Leadership and consultancy.
- Education, training and development.
- Practice development linked to research and evaluation.

In a study of role models, Donaldson and Carter (2005) found that students encountered both good and bad models. They found that undergraduate students were keen to stress the importance of good role models whose competence they could observe and practise, and receive constructive feedback on, so that they were able to develop their own competence and skill set, and thereby also their self-confidence.

Frameworks and approaches to practice teaching

Well-established models or frameworks for supervising learning are available for practice teachers to choose from for a more systematic approach to practice teaching. Models or frameworks are usually derived from empirical studies. For instance, the model for skill development for nurses advocated by Benner (2001), which comprises learning from being a novice to becoming an expert in the long term, was derived from a qualitative study in the 1980s in the USA. 'Approaches' to an activity, on the other hand, do not usually signify empirical derivation, but are based instead on the knowledge and experience of well-informed professionals in the field.

Consequently, a model comprises key components or steps for performing the task, and a well-used and tested model can mature into a more reliable framework to enable the practical application of various components (or steps) in a model.

The model of skills acquisition identified by Benner (2001), for instance, comprises being a 'novice' in specific skills at the beginning of one's professional career, and then progressing to become an advanced beginner, then competent, proficient and eventually an 'expert', in sequence. A simple illustration of how Benner's model of skills acquisition applies to the registrant acquiring critical-care nursing skills, for instance, is as follows:

- Novice: as a newly qualified nurse, able to perform generic nursing interventions based on evidence.
- Advanced beginner: performs certain specific critical care skills.
- Competent: able to use expanded role skills such as administering intravenous injections and blood-gas monitoring tasks safely and effectively.
- Proficient: performs the above activities efficiently and with a more extensive repertoire of theoretical knowledge.
- Expert: aware of numerous empirical studies in all aspects of critical care and able to engage in research as appropriate.

As models of practice teaching are as yet not adequately documented, the practice teacher can choose from and utilise the various general models and approaches to teaching, learning and assessment that are available. (Students' approaches to learning are discussed in Chapter 3 of this book.) It is imperative that the use of these models is underpinned by acceptance, genuineness and empathy, which are also essential components of 'helping' (and counselling) relationships (Rogers and Freiberg, 1994). However, counselling is a specialised and more complex process than supervision, and therefore supervision sessions must not be interpreted as counselling.

Models of supervision can be derived from various other fields such as dissertation supervision and clinical supervision. In the context of supervising doctoral students working on their research dissertations, Gatfield and Alpert (2002) suggest that the approach to supervision utilised should be guided by the level of structure and the level of support that the supervisee needs. These are:

- A *laissez-faire approach* – for students who require little structure and little support.
- A *contractual approach* – for students who require a high degree of structure and support.
- A *pastoral approach* – for students who require a high degree of support but little structure.
- A *directorial approach* – for students who require a high degree of structure but less support.

Practice teachers might choose to select and use relevant approaches suggested by Gatfield and Alpert (2002). Alternatively they could choose from the four models of mentoring in school-teacher training identified by Kerry and Mayes (1995) as the colleagual model, counselling model, professional model and the process model.

Models generally imply an essential set of components that are organised in a specific way to form a framework for enabling the particular activity to be performed effectively. Some of the key models and approaches that mentors use for supporting learning as identified by Gopee (2008a) include the apprenticeship model, reflective practitioner, competence-based model and the team-based model.

Action point 2.2: Utilisation of models of student supervision

Consider a number of learners whose learning you have facilitated in healthcare settings during your career, and think of which healthcare profession courses the students were on. Consider whether different approaches, models or frameworks for supervision of learning were the most appropriate for different categories of learners, and if so which ones, and jot down your thoughts. Also indicate the reasons for using those particular models or approaches.

A model is of course useful if it can be used as a framework for action. However, most of these models are currently not frameworks in that they don't identify a set of components, but are instead generally empirically untested, and still at an early stage of development. They are however malleable and can be modified to guide practice.

Learning contracts

The laissez-faire approach to supervision advocated by Gatfield and Alpert (2002) may not be appropriate for the supervision of students on healthcare courses, but the more structured ones are, and can include the utilisation of learning contracts or learning agreements.

Furthermore, formal documentation of specific supervision interactions is necessary, as it represents evidence of their occurence (NMC, 2009d). Consequently it is appropriate to complete a learning agreement, akin to that presented in Box 2.1. The proceedings or outcomes of discussions between the practice teacher and their supervisees need to be documented for a variety of reasons, which include keeping a record of progress as well as plans for subsequent learning activities. These plans can be formalised as the learning agreement or learning contract.

A 'learning agreement' is defined by the RCN (2002: 20) as '... a vehicle for ensuring that the planning of learning experiences is a mutual undertaking between a learner and their helper, mentor or teacher, and often their peers. As a result of this process, the learner develops a sense of ownership and commitment to their plan'.

Box 2.1   A learning agreement

Name of student:

Placement dates:
from .... to ....

Cohort:

Practice teacher's name:

Learning needs The skills and knowledge I want to acquire	Objectives What do I want to have achieved by the end of the placement? (i.e. specific objectives)	Resources and strategies How will I learn, and who will help me? (i.e. learning strategies and resources)	Target date Date by which the objective will be achieved	Evidence of achievement What evidence can I present to show that I have achieved my intended learning?
1. ... 2. ... 3. ...				

Agreement at the start of the placement

Student's signature: Date:

Practice teacher's signature: Date:

Name of link teacher/practice education facilitator: Name of personal tutor:

Comments on progress with agreed objectives – at midpoint or another agreed interval

Student's signature: Date:

Practice teacher's signature: Date:

Comments on achievement of agreed objectives

Student's signature: Date:

Practice teacher's signature: Date:

The use of a learning agreement advocated by the RCN (2002), for instance, comprises similar features to a learning contract, but is intended to be a more mutual and trusting agreement, and therefore might not include the signatures of those involved, nor strict 'achieve by' dates. It is a peer-assisting collaborative product, in which both parties are responsible for their decisions, and is therefore also less binding. The learning contract is a more definitive document that calls for accountability and is more legally binding. Naturally students need to give plenty of thought to the nature of the placement before identifying the objectives to be achieved.

Action point 2.3: The learning agreement

Consider any subsequent actions that the two parties could take after they have signed the learning agreement. What might these be?

The learning agreement comprises documentation regarding the student's learning under the practice teacher's supervision. In response to Action Point 2.3 you might have felt that the items in the agreement needed to be regularly visited as it is a live document and constantly reviewed to monitor the student's progress with its content, or only reviewed on the 'target date', i.e. how far the learning objectives in the learning agreement have been achieved.

Learning agreements might be viewed by some as unnecessary because the competencies to be achieved during the placement are already identified in a student's placement competencies booklet. Use of learning agreements is, however, based on andragogical approaches to teaching and learning, and therefore affords students further space to consider additional competencies that they might choose to learn in that particular (and related) field of practice, based on their own personal interests and aspirations.

The benefits of learning contracts include an improvement in student attendance at lectures and student performance in assessments, as found by Ghazi and Henshaw (1998), for instance, and in contributing to the achievement of module aims (Bailey and Tuohy, 2009).

The practice teacher's working relationship with post-qualifying students and mentors

Many components of the supervision of the pre-registration and post-qualifying students are similar in that a relationship has to be established initially and objectives identified, except the latter starts the contact using substantial professional knowledge and competence in the same or associated areas, and the competencies they have to achieve are those of specialist or advanced practice.

The NMC's (2008a) outcome for practice teachers includes practice teachers supporting mentors' and other registrants' learning. This reflects another dimension of the role that requires an effective working relationship.

Instances of when healthcare professionals might need support are, for instance, when a registrant has only recently completed a mentor preparation course, and needs preceptorship in the components of their role. Another instance is for peer-support e.g. if the practice teacher feels the need to discuss a certain situation with a colleague prior to making a decision about their mentee.

Managing inter-professional relationships

Each healthcare profession has already had its identity defined by its professional associations (e.g. the Chartered Society of Physiotherapy), and their regulatory body such as the Health Professions Council (HPC). The latter also identifies the 'Standards of Proficiency' for each healthcare profession. No doubt there are core elements to all healthcare professions that are largely dictated by their employers, e.g. infection-control processes, cardiac-arrest teams, moving and handling techniques, health and safety procedures, and development and performance review mechanisms.

As specialist and advanced practitioner roles are often multi-professional, a working relationship also needs to be established with members of other healthcare profession teams. For instance, a school nurse might work with social workers, schoolteachers, general practitioners, and so on, and one of their skills will be the ability to work collaboratively, which is based on using negotiation skills.

Working and learning inter-professionally

Healthcare professionals provide care and treatment for patients and service users as uni-, multi- or inter-professional teams. Different approaches to working with other healthcare professionals include:

- Multi-professional working – involves clinical interventions by health profession teams by virtue of medical referral of the patient/service user to the profession.
- Inter-professional working – refers to the above, but signifies appropriate levels of communication and collaboration between the healthcare professions.
- Trans-professional working – signifies more cohesive team working that also endeavours to eliminate or reduce the duplication of activities by different health-care professionals (e.g. single assessment process for older people – DH, 2007b).

The different approaches to working by members and teams of healthcare professionals all aim to restore the patient's or service user's health, which lends itself to inter-professional learning, i.e. healthcare professionals of different groups learning about each other, and from each other, which is also discussed in Chapter 3. Research on inter-professional education (IPE) reveals that it results in increased inter-professional collaboration that in turn results in co-ordinated and effective care and treatment (e.g. RCN, 2007a; Hammick et al., 2008). Some of these studies (e.g. Freeth et al., 2005) also highlight issues related to IPE which predominantly revolve around the way university courses and modules are delivered – as is also evidenced in Chapter 3.

Potential relationship problems in practice teaching

Arnold and Boggs (2003) identify the 'bridges' and the 'barriers' that can affect nurse–patient relationships. Barriers, if they occur, would result in an ineffective relationship and consequently negative outcomes. Despite the endeavours of facilitators of learning and their students, an effective working relationship could possibly still not materialise, and even when formed, can still break down. Problems and issues might arise, differences in views could surface and may even result in conflict situations. There can be a number of reasons for a working relationship not being established between practice teacher and student, which are now examined.

Relationship problems in clinical situations

Thus situations could arise when the practice teacher–student relationship is not functioning as effectively as it could, and there can be disagreement between different professional groups, or between practice teachers and their line managers regarding the channelling of resources, for instance, or friction between peers, or related to the transfer or discharge of patients. There can be disagreement regarding the communication of highly sensitive condition-related information, such as child abuse, to clients, relatives or students; or occasional aggressive outbursts by outsiders. Such strong disagreements can take the form of an actual conflict situation, which can be resolved by systematic problem-solving methods, or by utilising known ways of managing conflict effectively.

Action point 2.4: Dealing with difficult situations in facilitating learning and assessing students

1   Think of, and make notes on, all the probable problems you might encounter when facilitating learning or assessing student competence in your clinical setting.
2   Take one of the more difficult problems, and with one or two peers, identify and make notes on the pre-emptive actions that could have been taken to avert the issue, and the options available for resolving it.

When dealing with difficult situations in teaching and assessing students, the likely outcomes depend to a large extent on the practice teacher's leadership and accountability, which are examined later in this book. Moseley and Davies (2008) explored aspects that mentors find difficult to deal with, and concluded that in addition to cognitive or intellectual problems, mentors can find certain inter-personal and organisational factors difficult as well. These difficulties are related to:

- Staff attitudes.
- Students' level of preparation/skill.
- Number of students allocated to the clinical setting.

- Skill mix.
- Time availability.
- Number of shifts the mentor works with students.
- Students' timekeeping.
- Mentors' own preparation.
- Each student's personality.

The cognitive and intellectual factors that learning facilitators could find difficult related to developing effective relationships include integrating students into practice, providing constructive feedback to students, serving as a role model, assessing students, creating a learning environment and keeping up to date with students' programmes of study (Moseley and Davies, 2008).

Competing challenges and conflicts in practice settings

Following on from Phillips et al's (2000) and Nettleton and Bray's (2008) findings that learning facilitators fulfil their learning support role as one of many roles that compete for their time, there is a danger that they could experience role conflict. The different categories of roles fulfilled by practice teachers are clinician, teacher, leader/manager and researcher, or the dimensions (of NHS posts) identified in the *NHS KSF* (DH, 2004a), as noted in Chapter 1. Additionally, they are likely to engage in administrative work including the documentation of patient progress, being a line manager and/or shift manager, auditing, performing counselling or helping roles, being a keyworker, and undertaking various other activities.

Managing conflict

Working relationships are constructed over time, and they need to be maintained if the objectives of the relationship are to be achieved. However, it is important to recognise that relationships can break down if the goals, beliefs and values of the two parties are substantially different, and a lack of rapport prevails, or it never forms in the first place. Practice teachers' years of experience of working as specialist or advanced practitioners are likely to have included managerial activities, and thus resolving conflicts as they arise.

Causes of conflict in clinical settings

As it is a new role with no exact precedence, case studies and examples of practice teacher conflict are scarce. Conflicts that could arise include the general human-relations disjunctions that can occur between different healthcare profession groups, and within different domains of practice teaching identified by the NMC in relation to learning and assessment in practice settings, as noted by Nettleton and Bray (2008), for example, between the domains facilitating learning and the assessment of competencies. Conflict is defined by Sullivan and Decker (2009: 163) as 'the consequence of real or perceived differences in mutually exclusive goals, values, ideas, attitudes, beliefs, feelings or actions'.

Action point 2.5: Potential sources of staff conflict in practice teaching

Think of the practice teacher's role in the context of the eight NMC 'domains' for supporting learning, and that of the dimensions of the *NHS KSF* (DH, 2004a), and consider the likely areas, and some specific examples, of conflict situations that practice teachers might encounter either with colleagues or with pre-registration or post-qualifying students. Consider also other standards that the practice teacher might have to achieve in their specialist or advanced practice role.

On exploring conflict situations that might occur in practice teaching, based on other learning-support roles, it is possible to identify those that might include a lack of rapport between the two individuals, a personality clash, differences in perceptions of their roles and responsibilities, and each party's values and beliefs about healthcare and their roles. It could be due to technical reasons such as the student not being able to be punctual due to domestic constraints, or transport problems because the placement area is some distance away from the student's abode. Alternatively the practice teacher might be called upon to fulfil other clinical roles frequently or may have to work a different shift to the student's, due to day-to-day staffing requirements. In these circumstances, either party could perceive the other as being less committed to the relationship.

Another cause of conflict between individuals could well ensue from the practice teacher's continual interaction with various healthcare professionals in the day-to-day provision of healthcare in various departments, and having to make numerous decisions at work, some of which may not be agreeable to all the parties or individuals who are directly or indirectly affected by them. There are also various subcultures in different teams as influential individuals exhort others to think and work in particular ways.

The sort of conflict that a practice teacher might experience could be between themselves, i.e. their own values and goals for their patients, and possibly:

- their student
- social-care services
- the medical consultant
- general practitioners
- the trust's managers.

The managerial role of RNs includes being aware of problematic situations and occurrences that could surface in the course of their normal day-to-day duties, and they need to be able to foresee and avert these, or have a plan of action to resolve them if they occur. In response to Action Point 2.5, you should have been able to think of a few examples of sources of conflict that the practice teacher could countenance. The practice teacher can begin to act on potential or actual sources of conflict by starting to analyse its nature by recording them as follows.

Instances of potential sources of in practice teaching	How the practice teacher can deal with the conflict
Between the practice teacher and their student/other healthcare professionals:	
Between the practice teacher and social-care services:	
Between the practice teacher and the medical consultant:	
Between the practice teacher and the trust's managers/their own line manager:	
Between the practice teacher and general medical practitioners:	
Between the practice teacher's goals and corporate/departmental goals:	

With regard to conflict between students and their practice learning facilitators, Kantek and Gezer (2009), for instance, reported on a study of conflict management by students in Turkey, which unveiled that conflicts generally result in negative outcomes for students, who are generally aware of such outcomes beforehand, and can take proactive actions to avert or manage the conflict.

Despite the negative connotations of the concept, conflicts can also generate positive outcomes as they can also produce growth and new learning, depending on how they are managed. The likely negative outcomes of conflicts include the pervasion of a social atmosphere of suspicion and mistrust, a loss of motivation, a loss of confidence in the organisation, a resistance to teamwork, and individuals and groups becoming more egocentric. The general positive outcomes that could ensue from conflicts include an increased problem-solving ability through being forced to search for new approaches, developing negotiation skills, individuals' views being clarified and protocols initiated. Furthermore, both parties could learn new skills or gain new perspectives from each other. Conflicts are also an opportunity to identify CPD needs based on the actual issue. It can be a chance to network and make new professional acquaintances and to learn from the experience.

Strategies for resolving conflict

Various strategies that the two parties involved can take to manage the conflict are summarised in Box 2.2. A third party can be used as a catalyst. Thus, conflict can be resolved successfully if at least one party is clear about their goals and objectives, and more effectively if the two parties collaborate. If a third party is brought in to manage the conflict, then a systematic conflict resolution could result after analysing a variety of alternatives as positive opportunities, within an interactive and dynamic process. Constructively managed, such conflict can form the basis for changes in clinical practice.

Box 2.2 Strategies for managing conflict

Avoidance (lose–lose)– When neither party takes action to address the problem, and therefore no settlement is jointly reached.

Competition (lose–lose)– A strategy used by both parties in their endeavour to gain substantially better outcomes for themselves than for the other party, and a settlement is difficult to reach.

Confrontation– The problem is openly and vociferously discussed by all the parties involved.

Negotiation – The conflicting parties discuss the issues and give-and-take on particular elements.

Win–lose – One party wins, and the other loses.

Forcing – A senior member of staff issues orders on what the outcome of the conflict is to be, and may please one party or neither.

Smoothing – When differences are downplayed, minor areas of agreement are used as an end to the conflict.

Accommodation – One party makes disproportionate demands on the requirements for settling the conflict, and the other party gives in to a large extent.

Partisan choice – Attending to the needs of only one party.

Collaboration (win–win) – A joint-welfare strategy in which there is an endeavour to meet the needs and goals of both parties adequately.

A case study identifying an instance of conflict in the practice teacher role follows.

Case study

Leanne is a recently appointed health visitor in the local Primary Care Trust. She is on a permanent contract, with no probationary period, which is mainly because she has worked as a health visitor in another part of the country, and because the trust needed to appoint three health visitors quite quickly to be able to meet the local population's healthcare needs. Leanne was allocated to Jo as her preceptor to guide her through the trust's induction package of competencies for new appointees, and also because Leanne indicated that in her previous job, unlike the current allocated population area of service users, she had covered a different population involving high unemployment and crime.

Jo soon discovered that although Leanne is very fluent, her health-visiting clinical skills were suspect in many ways, and two months after starting in the post,

(Continued)

(Continued)

Leanne has not shown any inclination to allow Jo to observe her carry out any clinical interventions. Obviously, therefore, Jo could not sign off the competencies in the induction pack as having been achieved, nor allocate Leanne to attend to any of the clientele on her own. Leanne soon informed her union that she felt she was being bullied and unnecessarily closely observed. Jo informed her line manager that Leanne should be allocated to another practice teacher, as there was a lack of rapport between them, and that she was falling behind with her own work. However, on advice from her line manager, Jo wrote a letter to Leanne indicating her concerns about the lack of progress with the competencies in the induction pack. On receipt of the letter, Leanne responded via a verbally abusive telephone call to Jo, and stated that her husband who worked in a human-resources department in another organisation had said that the letter was in breach of employment regulations.

The above case study reflects interpersonal conflict situation, and potentially one between a recent employee and the employing trust. Jo's line manager could select from the strategies for managing conflict (identified in Box 2.2) to resolve the conflict situation between Leanne and Jo. At some point the line manager may have to decide to invoke the trust's disciplinary procedure if there is still no evidence of clinical competence.

Practice teachers can draw on the principles of conflict management just outlined, treat them as challenges that offer opportunities for learning from events, and then determine the stance and route that they want to take to avert or resolve conflict. This can be facilitated through clinical supervision, or with an appropriate colleague acting as a referee.

Where issues do arise, either in the form of latent or open conflict between peers, or with the healthcare professional's line manager or students, an open-minded approach needs to be taken to explore them, as further beneficial outcomes could ensue from differences in perception.

Conclusion

Chapter 2 has explored how working relationships are formed, maintained and managed between individuals and between students and their learning supervisors, specifically with regard to practice teaching. How students build relationships in different learning environments was explored, which by nature incorporates the dynamics of inter-professional working and inter-professional learning and education. Issues related to effective working relationships were also explored, as well as how they could be resolved or averted. To do this, the chapter explored:

- The reasons for healthcare professionals developing and establishing working relationships with a range of individuals, including patients and service users, other healthcare professionals, and healthcare students of course.

- The nature and dynamics of interpersonal relationships in general, and interpersonal communication and psychosocial development throughout life.
- How professional working relationships are formed between learning facilitators in the clinical setting and their students (pre-registration and post-qualifying), and with patients or service users, and how students initiate and build relationships in different learning environments, so as to identify the fundamental principles of relationship formation, with learning facilitators and students.
- Frameworks and approaches that practice teachers draw on to develop, establish and manage working relationships effectively with pre-registration and post-qualifying students, with mentors and other registrants who support their learning.
- How professional and inter-professional relationships are maintained and managed, and how they enable inter-professional working and learning.
- Potential problematic situations, especially the likelihood of interpersonal conflict, and how these can be averted or resolved, should they arise.

Establishing effective working relationships with students and peers is a mutually beneficial feature of the practice teacher's capabilities which needs to be maintained throughout students' practice placements, and beyond. Chapter 3 will focus on facilitating the learning of clinical skills for students on generic, and on specialist and advanced practice courses, by exploring the teaching and learning relationship in the supervision of practice learning for students on SPQ and ANP programmes.

3

Facilitating the Learning of Specialist and Advanced Clinical Practice

Introduction

Having examined the scope of the practice teacher role, and then ways of establishing and managing effective working relationships as a practice teacher so far, the third chapter of this book focuses on how practice teachers facilitate learning for students to enable them to acquire specialist or advanced practice knowledge and competence. It particularly focuses on the facilitation and supervision of practice learning for students on SPQ and ANP programmes, acknowledging the healthcare professionals' existing expertise in facilitating learning as a registrant, and possibly as a mentor.

Chapter outcomes

On completion of this chapter you should be able to:

1 Clearly distinguish between the concepts facilitation of learning and teaching, explain ways in which andragogical approaches, and other contemporary models and concepts of teaching and learning, can be applied to students' learning.
2 Critically evaluate how the practice teacher facilitates effective learning for students in clinical settings, including enabling students to access interprofessional learning opportunities and managing obstacles to learning.
3 Examine ways in which the practice teacher facilitates learning specialist and advanced practice knowledge and competence, and enables students to achieve standards of proficiency.
4 Identify the practice teacher's role in academic work through supporting learning across practice and academic environments, their contribution to curriculum planning for nurse education and in students' learning at different academic levels.

Teaching or facilitating learning

This section starts by identifying the range of personnel who teach specialist and advanced practice students in even one clinical specialist area, and then explores whether practice teachers should 'teach' their students, or 'facilitate' their learning. The application of andragogical approaches to learning follows.

Who teaches specialist and advanced practice students?

The facilitation of learning for specialist and advanced practice students is undertaken predominantly by practice teachers in the clinical setting, although it is fully recognised that they also gain knowledge and develop competence by working with a range of other healthcare and social-care professionals. Depending on the complexity of the clinical specialism and the module they are studying for, these other healthcare professionals can include medical consultants, pharmacists, pathology laboratory technicians, consultants in allied health professions and visiting speakers.

Specialist and advanced practice students are taught in practice as well as academic settings, and the facilitators of learning must therefore themselves be specialist or advanced practice professionals. Trudigan (2000) reports, for instance, on how she successfully combines her specialist practice role with her clinical educator role in her work in tissue viability, with both practice development and CPD components. Other academic staff who specialist or advanced practice students can learn from include PEFs and lecturer–practitioners, whose roles were identified in Chapter 1.

Should the practice teacher teach or facilitate learning?

Components of professional learning

The fundamental principles and methods of teaching are well documented in various books (e.g. Curzon, 2003; Gopee, 2008a). The professional knowledge and competence that students acquire under the supervision of the practice teacher, as for most other forms of professional learning programmes, consist of learning in three domains: knowledge, skills and 'attitude'. Bloom (1956) identified these three domains of learning as cognitive, psychomotor and affective domains, respectively.

Other authors have classified domains of learning differently. Gagne (1983) identified five domains: motor skills, verbal information, intellectual skills, cognitive strategies and attitudes. More recently, Rogers (2002), for instance, has suggested the mnemonic KUSAB to indicate five domains of learning: knowledge, understanding, skills, attitudes and behaviour.

Action point 3.1: Teaching or facilitating learning

Over time, the notion of teaching has evolved in the direction of the concept of the facilitation of learning, especially in the context of adult education.

Consider and make notes on what the two notions of teaching and facilitating learning signify to you in the context of general adult education, i.e. education or learning in general post-compulsory education. What do you feel are the differences? Then consider what teaching and facilitating learning signify in the context of pre- and post-qualifying learning in the healthcare professions.

You either know already or now realise after Action Point 3.1 that the facilitation of learning is a different concept from teaching, in that the latter usually implies the face-to-face imparting of knowledge and comprehension, and analysis of specific topic areas. Facilitating learning shifts the focus from the teacher to the student's learning requirements and approaches. Whilst there can be a complete match between the areas that the teacher wishes to teach and those that the student wishes to learn, this is difficult to know without asking the learner. It shifts thinking from the teacher imparting knowledge to students finding out for themselves, i.e. student-centred learning, which in turn enables a better retention of knowledge and understanding.

The verb facilitate is based in the French word *facile*, which literally means easy, and therefore to facilitate something means to make it easy. Beyond being a verb, the facilitation of learning is a concept in its own right, and a concept analysis of 'facilitation of learning' by Cross (1996), for instance, revealed that the term is used in several contexts, including physiological, educational, counselling/psychotherapy, social and theological. The analysis then identifies the defining attributes of the concept *facilitation* as a means of enabling change, in a climate for learning incorporating mutual trust, acceptance and respect. It includes student-centred, negotiated and collaborative learning. The antecedents of facilitating learning relate to the facilitator qualities, namely realness, caring and empathy, and access to a learning situation and the effects of motivation and social influences. The consequences of effective facilitation are reciprocal change (learning and understanding), reciprocal feedback and increased independence.

Rogers (2007) explores facets of the concept of the facilitation of learning, and suggests that it is a vital tool for helping adults to learn, and indicates that it is made up of several components, especially in the way particular groups need to be managed to ensure particular aims of the curriculum are achieved by the end of the session. However, one of the most influential proponents of the paradigm shift from teaching to the facilitation of learning is Carl Rogers (Rogers and Freiberg, 1994) who drew on his expertise in counselling and made landmark suggestions on how the fundamental principles of counselling can be applied effectively to the education of adult students. In particular, the 'conditions' required to form a working relationship that were discussed in Chapter 2 of this book are specifically pertinent.

The prevalence and influence of andragogical approaches

In education in general, two overarching broad approaches to teaching and learning prevail – the andragogical approach and the pedagogical approach. The andragogical approach is mostly utilised in the adult education arena, but can also be usefully applied to student learning in the post-compulsory sector.

Andragogical approaches to teaching and learning have been researched and well documented over the years, and therefore also represent an example of evidence-based teaching. Mezirow (1981), for instance, has researched for almost three decades how adults learn, and concludes that andragogy refers to self-directed learning which is undertaken in the form of courses of various durations, from half-day study days to full certificate-, diploma- or degree-awarding courses.

Mezirow and other researchers note there are differences in the way adults approach learning, as opposed to how children do so. Opposite to andragogy is pedagogy which refers to an approach that encompasses more direct imparting of knowledge, skills and attitude, akin to when teaching small children, but also applies to adults in, for instance, instructing them how to perform a skill such as how to drive, or how to deal with an emergency. Rogers (2002) identifies the characteristics of adult learners as adults who:

- are in a continuing process of growth
- bring with them a package of experience and values
- come to learning with intentions
- bring expectations about the learning process
- have competing interests
- have their own set patterns of learning.

Later theories and concepts that have emerged from research in teaching, learning and education encompass various different approaches to learning, including work-based or practice-based learning, which the practice teacher can adopt and utilise in their teaching as appropriate.

Furthermore, Rogers (2002) suggests that education is a planned learning opportunity which one party provides in relation to agreed objectives. He also suggests that the characteristics of education are that it is a process that is sequential and cumulative, is provided in accordance with chosen general principles and is in certain ways complete.

The practice teacher by virtue of this role operates in a medium that warrants the use of andragogical approaches as their supervisees are qualified, adult and experienced professionals on specialist or advanced practice programmes, or undergraduate healthcare profession students.

Contemporary theories and approaches to teaching and learning – an overview

In addition to andragogigal approaches, various models and theories of teaching and learning are available for practice teachers to choose from and utilise.

Models of teaching and learning

Joyce et al. (2009) explored models of teaching and learning that can be implemented in higher education, and suggested that there are models that are formal and well structured, whilst others are still emerging. They grouped the known models under four 'families of models' of teaching and learning, as briefly cited in Box 3.1. The 'families of models' presented in Box 3.1 are not in any particular order, nor does any new model or approach have to conform rigidly to one family of models or another. Rogers (2002) and Rogers (2007) categorise these approaches to teaching and learning in slightly different ways. However, contemporarily, when applied to educating healthcare professionals, all these models of teaching and learning need to take into account the influence and prevalence of andragogical approaches.

Box 3.1   'Families of models' of teaching and learning

Personal models	non-directive teaching, and learning as self-actualisation, e.g. experiential learning; and reflective practice
Behavioural models	e.g. social-learning theory; simulation-based learning
Social models	e.g. problem-based learning; role-playing; and peer-supported learning
Information-processing model	e.g. cognitive development; advanced organisers

The various foundational educational concepts and frameworks that have evolved since the advent of andragogy (adult education) have emerged predominantly from educational research with various groups of students and learners, and those explored in this chapter include:

- experiential learning
- reflective practice
- work-based learning and social-learning theory
- simulation-based learning
- problem-based learning
- peer-supported learning
- e-learning and blended learning.

Exploration of these theories is followed by a discussion on various approaches to learning that have also evolved, such as deep, surface and strategic learning. The concepts discussed are also derived from contemporary themes presented at national and international healthcare profession education conferences such as Net2009, the RCN Education Forum and RCN International Nursing Research, as well as other contemporary literature on the topic areas.

Other related and overlapping associated concepts that need further or ongoing research, and are discussed elsewhere in this book, include inter-professional learning, diversity and equality in education, 'fitness for practice' related to professional learning, and practice settings as learning environments. The practice teacher will have encountered a number of these concepts during courses that they have previously attended, or from their usual professional development readings. The next section presents a brief overview of contemporary concepts associated with learning in healthcare professions – they generally follow the order in which they are identified in Box 3.1

Experiential learning

The concept experiential learning refers to 'learning by doing', that is by experiencing novel activities and situations, and gaining insights or developing new skills by engaging with those situations and opportunities. Kolb (1984: 21) suggests that experiential learning comprises learning from 'here and now concrete experiences'. Experiential learning is a particularly useful means of learning clinical skills and to observe the effects of clinical interventions and decisions. These situations and learning opportunities can be structured into learning programmes, or can be based on incidental learning. To benefit fully from experiences of situations and opportunities just discussed, the individual needs to engage in structured reflection.

Reflective practice

Based on the principles of learning advocated by several including Kolb (1984) and Boud et al. (1985), reflective practice is well documented as a means of learning from day-to-day 'critical incidents', that is from situations that materialise during the course of the healthcare professional's normal work activities. Many day-to-day activities, whether they are routine or unusual, can therefore present as potential learning situations.

By exploring these incidents against the backdrop of existing published knowledge and experience in the field, new learning can ensue, and new ideas and solutions be generated.

Typically, reflective practice involves:

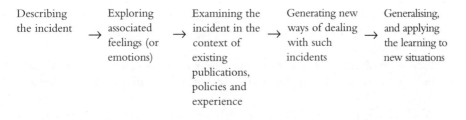

Describing the incident → Exploring associated feelings (or emotions) → Examining the incident in the context of existing publications, policies and experience → Generating new ways of dealing with such incidents → Generalising, and applying the learning to new situations

This method of learning therefore can enable the individual to develop new theories from professional practice situations, which can then be applied to similar situations when they recur.

All components of the sequence of reflection just described are important, but particularly so is the literature context, as well as the learning that emerges from it. However, any ensuing theory will need subsequent empirical testing to ascertain its validity and applicability. Healthcare professionals can then write reflective accounts of learning, and keep them in their personal and professional portfolios. If required as part of a course that the student is on, or as evidence of CPD, selected sections of the portfolio can be submitted for assessment. However, if the reflection is on a critical incident stemming from poor clinical practice, then the individual has a duty to take appropriate action, and the reflective account will need to comply with the rules of confidentiality.

Johns (1994) evaluated the effects of reflective practice as a means of 'professional supervision' of nursing colleagues, and demonstrated that it is an effective method of enabling healthcare professionals to learn in their new roles. Thus, in healthcare, reflective practice, that is learning from practice situations, is a useful conduit for developing new knowledge, and is a key component of personal and professional portfolios.

Manning et al. (2009: 176) explored the use of reflective groups for adult branch pre-registration students whilst they were undertaking practice placements, and found that group reflection sessions 'helped them to cope with the demands of the clinical environment and altered their perspectives on situations'. They report that students commented on the usefulness of the skills of facilitators in enabling them to see issues from a variety of perspectives and in guiding them to new insights, while also heeding confidentiality.

Work-based learning and social learning theory

Naturally a substantial proportion of learning that healthcare profession students undertake is achieved by observing skilled healthcare professionals performing clinical interventions in clinical settings, which they subsequently perform under the supervision of the practice teacher or another specialist. The notion of learning by observing experts in action in clinical settings is consistent with the concept of work-based learning, which can also be closely associated with 'social learning theory' (SLT).

Bandura (1977) is well known as a key advocate of SLT, which is based on observing the proficient or expert professional perform a skill, mentally rehearsing how the skill was performed step-by-step, participating in or performing the skill, gaining self and/or external reinforcement, and subsequently adopting the skill. Bandura refers to these processes of learning a skill as the four phases of learning: attentional processes, retention processes, the motor reproduction phase and motivational processes.

Positive reinforcement of learning constitutes a crucial component of SLT as it builds on previously advocated behaviourist-learning theories such as classical and operant conditioning.

Work-based learning (WBL) or 'practice-based learning' is defined by Flannagan et al. (2000: 363) as '… the bringing together of self-knowledge, expertise at work and formal knowledge. It takes a structured and learner-managed approach to maximising opportunities for learning and professional development in the workplace'. Dewar and Walker (1999) note that WBL is primarily concerned with the process of learning and with encouraging the individual to be explicit about how and what they learn so that their experiential learning may be assessed and accredited. These definitions emphasise some of the crucial components of WBL.

Work-based learning is very much a feature of health profession courses, and as the body responsible for approving the education programmes, the NMC (e.g. NMC, 2004a, 2004b) requires 50 per cent of the learning to be practice based, usually as practice placements.

There are obvious benefits in practice-based learning, hence the importance of practice placements for students on health-profession courses. Some of the strengths of WBL therefore are that it provides an opportunity to learn and acquire hands-on clinical skills, instils and builds self-confidence in performing clinical skills, involves multi-professional working, is grounded in the real world, in realistic situations with variable resources, is more patient-centred, allows learners to question rationales and the effects of clinical interventions, and is dynamic in that when the patient's condition changes treatment is adapted accordingly.

A study conducted by Moore and Bridger (2008) evaluated qualified nurses' engagement with WBL and its impact, and found that WBL enables learners to develop a range of intrapersonal, interpersonal and organisational skills, and is an effective tool for workforce development, advancing practice and 'tangibly enhanced patient care' (Foreword). The study report also includes a number of recommendations such as robust managerial support, as it also found that there are such organisational weaknesses as inconsistent appraisal and personal development plans mechanisms. However, there can be problems or issues related to WBL, and one way of identifying them is by a SWOT (strengths, weaknesses, opportunities and threats) analysis.

Action Point 3.2: Work-based learning – A SWOT analysis

Perform a SWOT analysis of the concept of work-based learning, or alternatively, you could choose to do a PESTLE (political, economical, social, technological, legal and ethical) analysis using a sheet of paper with four or six boxes, as appropriate.

The specialist or advanced practice nurse performing the skill therefore 'models' the skill, which implies that they need to be role models of clinical intervention, as healthcare professionals, as discussed in Chapters 2 and 8.

The likely weaknesses in WBL are a lack of time to reflect, having to work within resource constraints, and therefore achieving only minimum albeit safe standards rather than optimum standards, the learner might not appreciate the depth of theoretical knowledge required for relatively routine clinical procedures such as measuring blood pressure, and in mental health, the learner might not have the skill to be able to withdraw from a patient interaction situation. You are likely to have already identified potential opportunities and threats related to WBL that apply specifically to your area of professional practice.

A decade earlier, Guile and Young (1996) also identified issues with WBL such as behaviourist assumptions and a tendency towards reductionist approaches limiting WBL to 'know-how' rather than incorporating the related knowledge base, as well as the lack of comparability and equivalence between academic learning and WBL.

Simulation-based learning

Various reports of learning clinical skills by simulation have appeared recently. Joyce et al. (2009) suggest that teaching and learning by this method is a structured activity wherein the 'real world' is simulated inside a classroom (or skills laboratory for health-profession courses), and the concepts and tasks learnt are transferable to the real world. Marlow et al. (2008) report on simulation-based learning as an educational innovation whereupon they utilised 'technologically advanced manikins' in conjunction with health-problem scenarios to simulate real-life situations in their nurse education programme. Students on the programme indicated that they 'valued the opportunities to "practise safely" without the risk for repercussion to patients or themselves' (p. 188).

Moule et al. (2008) report on the outcomes of an NMC supported project on the simulated learning of clinical skills by adult and children-nursing student nurses, which was conducted at 13 universities. They explored student experiences and mentor views of the use of simulation for learning and concluded that simulation is positively received by both, and offered scope for inter-professional application and collaborative working between education providers and clinical staff.

Godson et al. (2007) report separately on the same project of simulation-based learning in which third-year student nurses were invited to teach clinical skills to first-year students. Evaluation of the project suggested that students favoured the strong peer-learning element in this form of teaching and learning. The implementation of the above-mentioned simulation-based learning projects was well designed. However, naturally learners learning clinical skills *ad hoc* from other learners in clinical settings must not be seen as actual teaching, as they might be incomplete, and there is always a danger of poor practice being imparted if students are not closely supervised.

Baker et al. (2008) explored learner and teacher reactions to 'simulation' in inter-professional education for patient-centred collaborative care. They found that simulation-based learning provided students with inter-professional activities that they saw as relevant for their future as practitioners. They concluded that 'inter-professional education through simulation offers a promising approach to preparing future healthcare professionals for the collaborative models of healthcare delivery being developed internationally' (p. 372).

Another slant to the concept is 'scenario-based learning' that Jones and Hardwick (2007), for instance, report is used in educational preparation programmes for paramedics teaching clinical skills.

Problem-based learning

As the term implies, problem-based learning (PBL) refers to learning by treating each new topic area, skill or situation as problematic, identifying various avenues and sources of learning such as literature and experts for learning about the component, acting on those ways of learning and discussing the learning in the presence of a facilitator. Lyons (2008) indicates that PBL requires students to work in small groups of six–eight students to identify and resolve real-life clinical problems through a combination of small-group processes and self-directed learning with the assistance of a facilitator who enables students to identify their learning needs and explore the application of new information to clinical settings.

Williams and Beattie (2008: 146) report on a systematic review of PBL which is utilised by clinicians as a method of clinical teaching in undergraduate healthcare programmes, and deduced that there is a paucity of evidence supporting or confirming the effectiveness of the application of PBL in clinical settings. The findings of the review therefore highlight current gaps in the PBL literature and therefore the need for further research into the role of PBL as a teaching strategy in the education of healthcare professionals.

However, on exploring second-year degree student nurses' use of PBL, Cooke and Moyle (2002) found that it promotes critical thinking, self-direction in learning, learning from peers, and the integration of a variety of knowledge. The practice teacher can utilise PBL in their role by enabling their supervisee's learning through methods that are consistent with the principles outlined in the definitions given above. For instance, if a student SCPHN encounters a situation where a new mother demonstrates apathy towards her newborn, then the practice teacher as a qualified SCPHN can take relevant action to ensure the safety of both, and that the baby's nutritional needs are being met, but for the supervisee's learning she may suggest to the latter that the situation can be treated as a 'problem', and the learner can explore and devise ways of resolving the problem by drawing on existing knowledge in published literature, policy documents and guidelines, and consulting relevant experts. The supervisee can work with another student or in a small group of peers on the SCPHN course in this pursuit.

Distler (2007: 58) reports on the implementation of PBL in an advanced practice curriculum in the USA, indicating that although more lecturers' time is required with PBL, 'the satisfaction and clinical confidence that students receive is well worth the effort', and rewarding for the academics as well.

Nonetheless, a database search of critically appraised research literature on PBL through the Cochrane library shows that that there is a dearth of 'high-quality' studies on the subject area. The systematic review that comes closest to the practice teacher's role is that by Smits et al. (2002) which explored the effectiveness of PBL in continuing medical education. They found no consistent evidence that PBL in continuing medical education was superior to other educational strategies in increasing doctors' knowledge and performance, although one of the high quality studies which compared problem-based with lecture-based learning showed more 'positive results' for PBL in terms of participants' knowledge, clinical reasoning and satisfaction.

Peer-supported learning and learning sets

The concept of peer-supported learning is also known by other similar terms with slightly different meanings, namely peer learning, buddying, human and social capital, and even peer reviews. Essentially peer-supported learning can be defined as learning that occurs in consultation and collaboration with peers in the same workplace or specialism, or students on the same course. The concept has been explored in various contexts. Classroom group work, workshops, seminar presentations and case conferences are some of the means by which individuals learn in the presence of, or from, each other. Small groups of student nurses or healthcare professionals on SPQ and ANP courses can arrange to meet regularly during practice placements, with or without an external facilitator, and learn about specific topic areas. One student can, for instance, explore and evaluate the role of community modern matrons and present their findings to a group of peers.

Course leaders tend to formalise peer-supported learning in the course curriculum in various ways, including by the use of 'action learning sets' (ALS), which McGill and Beatty (2001: 12) indicate comprise a group of individuals 'who have joined together expressly to work on a project, issue or problem which they intend to undertake, progress or solve'. They define action learning as 'a continuous process of learning and reflection, supported by colleagues, with an intention of getting things done' (p. 11). In the study of simulation-based learning reported by Marlow et al. (2008), they also indicate how as a project team successfully utilised the principles of ALS to work on their project. This suggests that ALS is not exclusively for students on a course, but can be usefully implemented in project-based activities. In fact, Graham (1995) identified a while back that action learning can be implemented in many forms of structured group learning with reflective practice incorporated as an underlying feature.

Graham and Partlow (2004) report on a study in which the use of 'co-operative learning' was implemented to help 'new' senior nurses develop their roles, and reflect on their acquisition of leadership skills and capability using a learning-set approach. They found that 'co-operative learning was an effective way of learning leadership skills, after the senior nurses in the study identified gaps in their knowledge and understanding of leadership. However, they found that, by exploring their life experiences through reflection and developing knowledge from theory as part of co-operative learning, they were able to construct strategies to help them manage their role in new and creative ways' (p. 459).

Peer learning also tends to be referred to as human and social capital (Gopee, 2002) in recognition of multifarious eventualities when students either organise learning in self-selected small groups or learn informally from each other in casual encounters.

Secomb (2008) conducted a systematic review of peer teaching and learning, and concluded that this mechanism increases students' confidence in clinical practice and improves learning in the psychomotor and cognitive domains. Negative aspects were also identified, which include poor student learning if either personalities or learning styles are not compatible.

E-learning and blended learning

With the continuing development of information and computer technology, increasingly either selected components, or whole higher-education programmes, are being offered in the distance learning mode as e-learning. This concept refers to learning through accessing learning materials made available electronically, mainly through computers, and as: (1) formal distance-learning courses accessed entirely on-line, and (2) informal access to knowledge through one's own volition.

The Quality Assurance Agency for Higher Education (QAA) (2008a: 1) identifies e-learning as a method of teaching and learning that 'looks at the adoption and expansion of the use of information and communications technology as part of the higher education learning experience'. As with distance learning, e-learning facilitates access to educational programmes without the constraints of time and place.

Various organisations, both those that have and those who have not traditionally been delivering open- and distance-learning programmes, have progressed to offer courses by e-learning. Examples of these are the Post-graduate Certificate in Academic Practice course offered by the Open University, a specialist healthcare profession course in Teenager and Young Adult with Cancer offered by Coventry University that successfully recruits and runs the course internationally entirely by e-learning, and a Master's in Business Administration courses.

However, generally assessment of clinical skills through e-learning programmes can be problematic, and needs to be organised locally. Some programmes combine e-learning with a reduced proportion of face-to-face teaching, which is then referred to as blended learning. Wakefield et al. (2008: 56) also note that there are different approaches to designing (or models of) blended learning programmes:

- Supplemental Model: retain traditional course structures, and support them with e-learning materials and activities.
- Replacement Model: a selection of face-to-face contact activities are replaced by e-learning activities and communication.
- Emporium Model: formal lectures are replaced by e-learning activities supported by open-access learning resources that actively encourage students to use enquiry-based learning strategies.
- Buffet Model: students are afforded flexible learning pathways allowing them to opt to engage with a range of learning environments and/or activities.

The QAA (2008a) acknowledges that e-learning is fast becoming firmly established as a core activity in many HEIs in the UK. Based on information gathered from institutional audits of HEIs in England and Northern Ireland during 2004 and 2006, the QAA concludes that, in general, the increased use of e-learning has been welcomed by students, but the need to obtain student feedback is seen as very important, and to take action as required.

Research on e-learning comparing specific e-learning programmes with other modes of programme delivery such as taught courses is currently limited. Reime et al. (2008) compared the use of e-learning versus lecture methods in teaching infection control to nursing students, and found that students were satisfied with both teaching approaches, and the e-learning programme was rated as good on design, academic content, and the integrated tests were motivating for their learning. They recommend that e-learning infrastructures have to be viewed as a resource in the same way as for lectures, and therefore also recommend the use of many different teaching methods to achieve the goals of the programme. It is obviously crucial though for students to be competent in the use of computers.

McVeigh (2009) explored the factors that may influence the utilisation of e-learning by nursing, midwifery and health-visiting students undertaking post-registration studies and found that students' perceptions of e-learning are positively influenced by its flexibility in time management, pace of learning, self-direction and widening access to information. McVeigh also identified the potential barriers related to e-learning as the individual preferences of students, levels of computer literacy, e-learning as being time consuming, competing with home-life elements and insufficient work-based support.

Research on e-learning and blended learning programmes therefore identified both the feasibility and the benefits of these two methods of programme delivery, and the potential problematic areas, which course designers need to be mindful of to ensure students learn at the appropriate academic levels as identified by the National Committee Inquiry into Higher Education (NCIHE) (1997) (Dearing Report) and the QAA (2008b), for instance. Good practice guidelines for implementing e-learning have been identified by various authorities, including the Higher Education Funding Council for England (2005) and the QAA (2008a).

Approaches to learning

In contrast to andragogical approaches to teaching and learning, Ramsden (2003) and Marton et al. (1997) are amongst recent educational researchers who have studied the approaches to learning that students choose to take when they enrol on a particular programme of study. For some short courses or modules, the student might choose the deep-learning approach and therefore actively engage with the subject area in depth and detail. On other programmes, they might select the surface approach, for example when listening to sales talks, and choose to merely become cognisant about the subject area without undertaking research and exploring the topic in great detail. For other programmes, wherein the student merely wishes to pass the module and gain a qualification, they might focus predominantly on the assessment requirements and channel their energies into this in particular. Biggs and Tang (2007) argue that those involved in teaching students on higher-education courses must ensure they are competent to motivate students to take the deep approach to learning.

In concluding this discussion on the more recent and innovative models and approaches to teaching and learning, the best source of evidence of their effectiveness is, of course, student evaluation of these strategies, and educational-research findings. As for research, Distler (2007), for instance, explored the development of critical thinking and clinical competence resulting from the implementation of student-centred and problem-based teaching strategies in an advanced practice nurse curriculum, and reported that even though more lecturer time is required, the clinical confidence that students gain from this method is very high, and it can also form the basis for innovations.

The practice teacher needs to be aware of many of these contemporary learning concepts as they are likely to be documented in, and to influence, the way pre-registration and specialist and advanced practice professional education programmes are delivered. Furthermore, as these concepts, theories and approaches are based on a number of research studies, such as those already cited in this chapter, they also form evidence-based teaching and education.

The practice teacher's role in the facilitation of learning

As discussed earlier in this chapter, one of the key roles of the practice teacher is to facilitate learning for students on healthcare and social care-profession education programmes, particularly during practice placements. This function includes utilising effective learning-facilitation skills within an optimal environment for learning and inter-professional education.

Effective learning facilitation skills

The facilitation and supervision of learning is identified as one of the key areas of activity for practice teachers. The NMC (2008a) identifies the outcomes for the practice teacher in relation to the facilitation of learning and creating an environment for learning as follows:

The facilitation of learning:

- enables students to relate theory to practice whilst developing critically reflective skills
- fosters professional growth and personal development by the use of effective communication and facilitation skills
- facilitates and develops the ethos of inter-professional learning and working.

Creating an environment for learning:

- enables students to access opportunities to learn and work within inter-professional teams
- initiates the creation of optimum learning environments for students at registration level and for those in education at a level beyond initial registration.
- works closely with others involved in education – in practice and academic settings – to adapt to change and inform curriculum development.

The key concepts inherent in these outcomes are:

- the integration of theory and practice
- reflective practice skills
- effective communication skills
- the facilitation of learning
- inter-professional learning and working
- optimum learning environments for pre- and post-qualifying students
- adapting to change
- communicating with academics to influence course curricula.

Each of these concepts is examined in substantial detail in different chapters where they are closely linked to particular components of the practice teacher role. Theory–practice integration is, for example, discussed in Chapter 7 in the context of the practice teacher's leadership, as is creating and maintaining an optimum environment for learning in clinical settings. Reflective-practice skills and facilitation of learning were explored in Chapter 3, and the communication and interpersonal skills required for establishing professional working relationships were explored in Chapter 2. Managing change is discussed in Chapter 4, inter-professional learning and the practice teacher's role in academic settings are examined later in this chapter.

Furthermore, it is also appropriate to note that the practice teacher's role includes teaching and assessing pre-registration students, who during their final placement have to be assessed and signed-off on a number of identified clinical skills that are inherent components of the NMC's (2004b) standards of proficiency. The NMC is then notified that a student is competent in these skills, which are mandatory requirements, for their name to be entered onto the NMC's register of qualified nurses.

Blocks to learning

Learning in both academic and clinical settings is fully planned and structured well in advance to ensure a fully beneficial learning experience for the student. However, unanticipated issues can surface and block learning. In managing learning, the practice teacher needs to take into account potential blocks to learning, such as the unavailability of various types of resources, the different academic levels that varions students are at in their programme of study, effective working and learning within inter-professional teams, learning in other healthcare and social-care professions, and fostering and facilitating professional growth and personal development.

The practice teacher will generally have devised a sketchy plan of clinical experiences for their student before the latter starts on placement, which is then structured fully soon after the initial meeting between student and practice teacher at the beginning of the placement. However, student learning can be marred by various factors, including unforeseen events. Research on general adult education has focused on inherent aspects such as access and the barriers to formal education for adults (e.g. McGivney, 1990).

Action point 3.3: Blocks to learning specialist or advanced practice skills

Based on your own professional experience and thoughts, make notes on what you feel are the factors that you consider can constitute obstacles to the learning of specialist or advanced practice clinical skills by your student in your work-place during practice placements.

The practice teacher's day-to-day schedule is replete with demands on their time, which can consequently delay or block learning. Blocks to learning can generally be categorised under four groups of factors:

- situational circumstances – e.g. access to the supervisor, staff shortages, distractions
- learning programme assignments requirements by the university – a disjunction between the outcomes that the university expects a student to achieve during the placement and the unavailability of appropriate clinical experiences
- student issues – e.g. a perceived lack of motivation, technical difficulties preventing the student from arriving on the placement on time
- personality and relationship issues – when one party projects disinterest and a lack of respect for the other, or when there are rapport problems.

Rogers (2002) discusses a number of factors that can block learning in adult education, with personality factors between student and teacher being one, while the learner's pre-existing knowledge of the subject, if that is erroneous or lacking in sufficient detail, is another.

Action point 3.4: Dealing with blocks to learning

Consider all the above discussions under the heading 'Blocks to learning' and make a list of those blocks to learning that most apply to your role as a practice teacher. Using the format below, itemise these in the left-hand column, and make notes in the right-hand column on how each block to learning can be managed, either by pre-empting them or as a problem to solve. You may wish to do the same in relation to learning generic clinical skills.

Blocks to learning	Actions that can be taken to pre-empt or problem-solve
Blocks to learning specialist or advanced practice skills	
Blocks to learning essential skills	

Individual clinical settings might each have their own particular facilities and constraints, and therefore factors that can block learning might also be closely linked to the availability of resources in the setting, both human and non-human. However, most healthcare trusts now have comprehensive facilities in terms of a library and include access to information technology for the effective facilitation of learning. The case study below illustrates an instance of blocks to learning and how these can be overcome.

Case study

Jen is a very experienced school nurse who started on the practice teacher course but dropped out two-thirds of the way through. She qualified as a school nurse almost ten years ago, when some of the current education theories and concepts were still in the early stages of being implemented. The main reason given for her dropping out of the course (indirectly) was that a number of the concepts being discussed were either new to Jen, or they were familiar sounding but she didn't feel she fully understood them. Jen felt that this was to do with the practice teacher course being at postgraduate level, and also felt that she was unlikely to be able to pass the course assignments, and would struggle to teach students on the school nursing specialist practice course during practice placements at this academic level.

However, at that point in time Jen also had some personal difficulties to contend with, and was off on sick leave for a number of weeks. On her to work, Jen and her learning supervisor met to explore the way forward with the practice teacher course. The course delivery for Jen's group had been completed by then, and consequently it was suggested that maybe Jen could shadow a qualified practice teacher prior to recommencing on the practice teacher course, so that she can gain some experience of the dynamics and nature of the interaction with specialist practice students. It was also suggested that the course director should perhaps hold pre-course interviews (albeit informally) where the concepts addressed during the course could be highlighted, so that prospective students could look some of them up in their own time prior to commencing on the course. Jen would be able to resume the practice teacher course when she wished to do so, and could draw on the university's writing skills department's help with her assignments as and when she wished to do so.

(Continued)

(Continued)

However, Jen's learning supervisor firmly believed that it was essential for all practice teacher students to shadow qualified practice teachers prior to starting on the course, as well as during it, to gain experience of this role, as being an experienced healthcare professional does not in itself constitute evidence of the ability to teach students on specialist education programmes anyway.

Inter-professional working and learning

Inter-professional working and learning in healthcare professions has been widely recommended for some time (e.g. DH, 1999; DH, 2008a; NMC, 2008a). In Chapter 2, the context of a working relationship between healthcare profession groups was explored and distinctions were made between inter-, multi- and trans-professional working.

In healthcare, inter-professional working is preferred to the other forms of input from different healthcare professions because it implies collaborative work between members of different healthcare professions who contribute to the health and wellbeing of the individual patient or service user. Such collaboration lends itself to learning from each other about patients' or service users' care and treatment. Inter-professional learning tends to imply informal and ad hoc learning whilst the term inter-professional education signifies the quest for knowledge and competence as part of a structured professional development programme.

Freeth et al's (2005: 17) definition of inter-professional education is widely accepted, and is also endorsed by the Centre for the Advancement of Inter-Professional Education (CAIPE), which is '… when two or more professions learn with, from and about each other to improve collaboration and the quality of care'. Effective inter-professional learning in university healthcare education programmes is structured within pre-registration undergraduate programmes through curricular activities based on case studies of patient journeys (or patient pathways) (e.g. DH, 2004c) through the healthcare system. Students explore situations in small working groups comprising students from a combination of healthcare professions, namely doctors, occupational therapists and, physiotherapists, and thereby gain other perspectives.

Inter-professional education

Recent research on the prevalence and scope of inter-professional learning suggests that it is beneficial in several ways. Clifton et al. (2006) explored the impact and effectiveness of IPE in primary care through a literature review, which revealed that IPE is generally enjoyed by students, may contribute to an improved knowledge and understanding of the roles and functions of the healthcare professionals involved, and may lead to more positive attitudes and perceptions of other healthcare professions. It also showed that there is strong policy commitment to IPE in the UK at both pre-qualifying and CPD levels.

However, the literature also suggests that IPE policies are based on the presumption that IPE leads to better clinical practice as indicated in self-reports, but none of the studies on the effectiveness of IPE programmes in primary care were rigorous, nor met the standards for a Cochrane review. Nonetheless, a subsequent systematic review concluded that IPE is generally well received as it enables learning the knowledge and skills necessary for collaborative practice (Hammick et al., 2008).

An extensive review of research on IPE was conducted by CAIPE (DH, 2007c), which included systematic reviews and experiences of IPE across the healthcare and social-care sector, which it concluded with a framework to inform good practice in IPE, for effective inter-professional collaboration, thereby improving the quality of patient care. The framework comprises several recommendations, including:

- professional bodies, sector skills councils, quality-assurance bodies, commissioners, education providers and employers working together to ensure that the quality of the inter-professional elements of healthcare, social care and children's services education programmes are monitored continually
- commissioners, education providers and employers ensuring that inter-professional education is mandatory and assessed within healthcare, social care and children's services and training programmes resulting in an award.
- stakeholders, together with CAIPE, should develop a national mechanism to recognise and reward organisations with a sustainable collaborative culture.

Facilitating the learning of specialist clinical skills or advanced practice

Having examined the concepts of teaching and learning and the practice teacher's role in the facilitation of learning, this section of the chapter explores facilitating the learning of specialist and advanced practice clinical skills in the context of the uniqueness of each specialist and advanced practice setting. New ways of working and their impact are then discussed, and how students can develop and achieve standards of proficiency.

The contexts of specialist and advanced practice, and their uniqueness

The current position regarding definitions and roles of specialist and advanced practitioners was explored in detail in Chapter 1. CNSs and ANPs are based in all clinical areas in the care and management of patients or service users with long-term conditions, or in acute- and primary care settings. In terms of facilitating learning in these settings, the practice teacher is the specialist or advanced practitioner. The SCPHN, for instance, is likely to be based in or attached to a primary care team in a health centre, or a GP practice. The role is fulfilled in a unique way as defined by the NMC (2009b).

For instance, the CNS based in a respiratory unit will normally be an expert in managing such conditions as asthma and chronic obstructive pulmonary disease, but they will also have a major role in teaching colleagues. Teaching can occur whilst performing a specialist clinical intervention, or in a teaching room at the unit, at the trust's post-graduate centre, or at the partner university.

Similarly, the emergency nurse practitioner is an advanced practitioner in an acute area. A CNS in a mental health care setting might be a mental health nurse who is a specialist in cognitive behaviour therapy or in the management of self-harm and might be based in a hospital or primary care centre but will work closely with allied healthcare and social-care professionals in the community.

Facilitating the achievement of specialist and advanced practice standards of proficiency

Specialist and advanced practice courses specific to different specialisms are offered at different universities and are available at undergraduate and post-graduate academic levels, depending on applicants' needs. As in pre-registration courses, the NMC (2008a) requires students on specialist and advanced practice courses to undertake 50 per cent of their learning in practice settings. During the practice part of the programme, students are assessed on specific practice outcomes adapted predominantly from the NMC's (2004a) standards of proficiency. Practice outcomes are also different based on the designation of the qualification that will be recorded on the NMC's register, for example an SCPHN in school nursing, as identified in Box 1.5 in Chapter 1. The NMC (2004a) details the outcomes of standards of proficiency for SCPHNs under four domains and ten principles, which are presented in Table 3.1.

Table 3.1   *SCPHN competency domains and principles*

Domain	Principle
Search for health needs	• Surveillance and assessment of the population's health and wellbeing
Stimulation of awareness of health needs	• Collaborative working for health and wellbeing • Working with, and for, communities to improve health and wellbeing
Influence on policies affecting health	• Developing health programmes and services and reducing inequalities • Policy and strategy development and implementation to improve health and wellbeing • Research and development to improve health and wellbeing
Facilitation of health-enhancing activities	• Promoting and protecting the population's health and wellbeing • Developing quality and risk management within an evaluative culture • Strategic leadership for health and wellbeing • Ethically managing self, people and resources to improve health and wellbeing

The outcomes or competencies under the domain 'Search for health needs' and the principle 'Surveillance and assessment of the population's health and wellbeing' are:

- collect and structure data and information on the health and wellbeing and related needs of a defined population
- analyse, interpret and communicate data and information on the health and wellbeing and related needs of a defined population
- develop and sustain relationships with groups and individuals with the aim of improving health and social wellbeing

- identify those individuals, families and groups who are at risk and in need of further support.
- undertake the screening of individuals and populations and respond appropriately to findings.

An initial formal discussion at the start of the practice placement is essential to ensure agreement on the competencies to be achieved, and to complete documentation, which in turn might incorporate a written learning contract, a concept that was discussed in Chapter 2.

The practice teacher and supervisee must continue to have discussions during the practice placement so as to monitor learning, but more importantly for the practice teacher to demonstrate an interest in the supervisee's progress with learning. An interim mid-placement formal discussion is also important to formally identify learning needs and subsequently, so that the competencies that have been achieved are signed off. Various components of the ways in which a practice teacher facilitates learning are identified in Box 3.2.

Box 3.2   The learning facilitation roles of the practice teacher

- Utilising teaching skills in both formal and informal settings.
- Identifying patient outcomes as ways in which specialist and advanced practice benefits patient and service user care.
- Applying theories of learning (e.g. reflective practice) to practice learning.
- Identifying suitable learning opportunities.
- Considering different levels of learning.
- Managing learning.
- Use of e-learning mechanisms.
- Teaching in academic settings.
- Fostering and facilitating professional growth and personal development.
- Integration of theory and practice.
- Facilitating the learning of specialist clinical skills in different practice settings, e.g. primary care, advanced emergency care, palliative care, long-term conditions.
- Facilitation of the achievement of specified standards of proficiency and practice outcomes.
- Working and learning within inter-professional teams.
- Creating optimum learning environments.
- Contributing to the curriculum development for appropriate courses.

However, Benner (2001) notes that skills are learned over a matter of time, on a spectrum which starts from being a novice to eventually becoming an expert, as briefly alluded to in Chapters 1 and 2. Specialist and advanced care practitioners (these terms were defined and differentiated from each other in Chapter 1) are generally at a much further stage than 'proficient' and are usually experts, depending on their post-qualifying experience.

The practice teacher's role in academic work

As specialist or advanced practitioners, practice teachers have a substantial educational role that extends to input into formal student-education programmes in academic settings, which is also advocated by the NMC (2008a). For example, under the leadership domain, this indicates that the practice teacher must 'demonstrate the ability to lead education in practice, working across practice and academic settings' (p. 56); and under 'Create an environment for learning', the practice teacher must work closely with others involved in education, in practice and academic settings, to adapt to change and inform curriculum development' (p. 55).

Supporting learning in academic environments

The practice teacher's role-set includes working with relevant healthcare academics. They might be invited to input quite substantially to course planning and delivery (i.e. lecturing), that is as both a member of the curriculum planning or review team of relevant post-qualifying courses, and in facilitating learning in some or substantial components of the programme.

Furthermore, as already indicated earlier on in this book, the practice teacher needs to be conversant with the curriculum of the course that their students are on. The practice teacher also engages in reporting issues related to practice placements. Moreover, the practice teacher may figure in academic settings in relation to their own annual update or triennial review as a practice teacher in the local register, as indicated by the NMC (2008a).

Thus the practice teacher's education role spans teaching in practice and in academic settings, and one way of doing this is through informing curriculum development. This role can be fulfilled by the practice teacher giving feedback and making suggestions to the HEI on relevant aspects of the specialist practice or pre-registration student's curriculum, or on issues related to supervision during a practice placement, or, as noted above, as a member of the curriculum planning team. The next section briefly examines how nurse education curricula are informed.

Nurse education curricula

The annual update study days for practice teachers normally include a session in which the technicalities and dynamics of the curriculum of the course that the practice teacher student is on, are explained. Curriculum planning takes time as the approaches taken, the content of the course, and so on, are discussed and agreed. As indicated earlier in this chapter, andragogical approaches to teaching and learning are one way of influencing the nature of the curriculum. However, more structured models of curricula reflecting the underpinning educational philosophy adopted need to be agreed before the course design can be started.

One of the most influential contemporary educational philosophies under-pinning course design is that advocated by Biggs and Tang (2007). They suggest an 'outcomes-based teaching and learning' approach to quality education (p. 6), and provide a framework for curriculum development, which they refer to as 'constructive alignment'. The framework is constructive in that it puts an emphasis on how learners construct knowledge, and alignment refers to a programme that states upfront the course aims, the intended learning outcomes, the teaching and learning activities, and the 'assessment tasks'. It comprises a student-centred curriculum that is informed by student feedback.

Quinn and Hughes (2007) identify a 'critical path' as the route taken to plan and deliver a course from the point in time when the course is an idea of either the HEI's academics or a course-purchaser organisation, to the point when the first intake of students starts. This involves the formation of a course planning team, unit writing, document writing, internal validation, document to panel, the full validation event, a response to validation conditions, which when addressed reaches the point when the first intake of students can start on the course. These stages are followed by various activities until the first intake of students completes the course, and it is finally evaluated as to its fitness for practice, purpose and award (NCIHE, 1997).

The QAA (2006), whose role includes auditing education programmes provided by HEIs in the UK, publishes various guidelines, which are usually available on its website. The curriculum also needs to consider and incorporate the QAA's (2008b) *Framework for Higher Education Qualifications in England, Wales and Northern Ireland*, which identifies qualification descriptors for unit and course outcomes for the different levels of learning that correspond with the student's first year at university as an undergraduate, their second year, third year, Master's level and doctorate level.

Various other factors influence the content and delivery of education programmes for healthcare professionals, which cover national and European policies and current research findings. Relevant recent healthcare and educational policy and guideline documents include:

- Chief Nursing Officer's *Essence of Care* series (e.g. DH, 2009b)
- *Modernising Nursing Careers: Setting the Direction* (DH, 2006a)
- Department of Health's *National Service Frameworks* (e.g. DH, 2001b)
- *NHS Knowledge and Skills Framework* (DH, 2004a)
- *NHS Improvement Plan: Putting People at the Heart of Public Services* (DH, 2004b)
- *The Framework for Higher Education Qualifications in England, Wales and Northern Ireland* (QAA, 2008b)
- *Standards of Proficiency for Pre-registration Nurse Education* (NMC, 2004b)
- *Towards a Framework for Post-registration Nursing Careers – consultation response report* (DH, 2008a).

Some policy publications are influenced by research reports conducted on behalf of regulatory bodies such as the NMC. For example, Longley et al's (2007) *Nursing: Towards 2015 – Alternative Scenarios for Healthcare, Nursing and Nurse Education in the UK in 2015* is a NMC-commissioned report on the future of pre-registration nurse education.

The publishers of the above-mentioned examples of policy documents that influence course planning for healthcare professions (i.e. the DH, QAA and NMC) are in fact some of the 'stakeholders', as they expect universities offering nurse education courses to comply with their guidelines and requirements. Stakeholders is a term that is used in this context to identify all parties that have an interest in the specific education programme, which is because the success or failure of the programme affects them in some way. In addition to the stakeholders already mentioned there are others including Strategic Health Authorities, local healthcare trusts, universities, students, and patients and service users. The RCN (2002) indicates that the key stakeholders for the practice element of nursing and midwifery programmes in practice placements are:

- students
- patients/clients cared for within all sectors where health care is provided
- the NHS and independent sector
- higher education institutions – staff such as personal tutors, programme directors, cohort leaders and subject/module/academic leaders/link lecturers
- service providers – these are part of the tripartite arrangements, with HEIs and the commissioning body, which should work together to enable students to achieve their registration (including the clinical team, mentors, lecturer-practitioners and PEFs)
- the commissioning bodies for education in England, Wales, Scotland and Northern Ireland.

Course design is also influenced by innovations in nurse education and research. A number of these innovations, many featuring evaluative studies, are publicised principally through nursing journals, some of which are incorporated within this book, while others are reported at appropriate national and international conferences.

Students learning at different academic levels

In the framework for higher education, the QAA (2008b) identifies 'qualification descriptors' for studying and assessment at different academic levels. Courses on specialist and advanced practice are increasingly offered at Master's level, and the QAA's guidelines comprise one model for discriminating between certificate, diploma, degree, Master's and doctorate level studies. The descriptors also comprise guidelines for learning in academic and clinical settings, as well as an assessment of knowledge and competence.

The QAA indicates, for instance, that holders of Master's level qualifications must be able to deal with 'complex issues both systematically and creatively', and demonstrate originality in the application of knowledge, in the use of self-direction, and in tackling and solving problems (p. 13).

The QAA's (2008b) 'descriptors' for qualifications at different academic levels cover from the first year of university studies to doctoral studies for a qualification such as Doctor of Philosophy (for the UK except Scotland) – see Box 5.1 in Chapter 5 for an example of a level descriptor for the third year of university degree level studies (level 6) in the context of differentiating between different academic levels of learning in the healthcare professions.

Conclusion

Chapter 3 has focused on the facilitation of the learning of clinical skills by students on generic, and on specialist and advanced practice courses, by initially considering the developmental framework and continuum identified by the NMC. It explored the teaching and learning relationship in the supervision of practice learning for students on SPQ and ANP programmes (NMC, 2008a) through to building on mentors' existing knowledge, competence and experience. Almost all of the theories discussed are extracted from research which identified their strengths as well as any of their problematic areas. This chapter thus examined:

- Contemporary paradigms in teaching and facilitating learning, including andra-gogical approaches.
- Relevant contemporary models of teaching and learning, namely reflective practice, experiential learning, work-based learning, simulation-based learning, problem-based learning, peer-supported learning, e-learning and blended learning; and approaches to learning.
- The practice teacher's role and competence in the effective facilitation of learning, blocks to learning, and working and learning interprofessionally.
- Facilitating students to learn and develop their specialist or advanced practice knowledge and clinical skills, and facilitating the achievement of specialist and advanced practice standards of proficiency.
- Practice teachers' role in academic work, including supporting learning across practice and academic environments, their contribution to curriculum planning for nurse education, and students learning at different academic levels.

Although the two activities of teaching and facilitating learning overlap in meaning, they comprise an indispensable feature of the practice teacher role. Chapter 4 will centre on the practice teacher's role in evidence-based practice (EBP), in the context of specialist or advanced practice and in practice development.

4

The Practice Teacher, Evidence-based Practice and Practice Development

Introduction

Having explored the scope of the practice teacher role – how the practice teacher establishes and manages effective working relationships, and facilitates the learning of specialist and advanced clinical practice skills – so far in this book, Chapter 4 centres on the practice teacher's role as an effective clinician in terms of being an evidence-based specialist or advanced practitioner, and a practice developer. Practice teachers as innovators and 'nurse entrepreneurs' are inherent concepts and activities that also involve disseminating innovative clinical practices, managing change and innovations, and the practice teacher's role as a 'researcher'.

Chapter outcomes

On completion of this chapter you should be able to:

1 Articulate analytically the practice teacher's role as an evidence-based practitioner, including knowledge of what EBP is, the reasons for and sources of EBP in the context of specialist and advanced practice.
2 Demonstrate an analytical knowledge of the practice teacher's role as a practice developer, that is of current perspectives on clinical practice development, and ensuring that particular professional learning needs are met in support of practice development.
3 Explore the practice teacher's role in research in relation to the utilisation of research findings, in engaging in applied research and in disseminating findings from research and innovative clinical practices.
4 Analytically recognise the value of new ways of working, ascertain the changes in established professional roles, manage change and innovations, and evaluate the effectiveness of practice development.

The practice teacher as evidence-based practitioner

Evidence-based practice figures widely in healthcare professions. It is a competency that is achieved during pre-registration programmes, is very much a central dimension of specialist and advanced practice, and is also an NMC outcome for learning facilitators such as mentors and practice teachers.

Evidence-based practice – definitions and a brief overview

The practice teacher as a specialist or advanced practitioner will already be cognisant of various elements of EBP. They will be aware that there are various definitions of EBP, such as that given by Melnyk and Fineout-Overholt (2005: 6) who identify EBP as: '... a problem-solving approach to clinical practice that integrates a systematic search for, and critical appraisal of, the most relevant evidence to answer a burning clinical question, one's own clinical expertise, and patient preferences and values'.

As for evidence-based nursing (EBN), Scott and McSherry (2009) explored the literature on key concepts that are inherent components of EBN in an endeavour to substantiate an operational definition of EBN for nurses to use in practice, and consequently synthesised a definition of EBN as 'an ongoing process by which evidence, nursing theory and the practitioners' expertise are critically evaluated and considered, in conjunction with patient involvement, to provide delivery of optimum nursing care for the individual' (p. 1089). They indicate, however, that for nurses to engage with and apply the evidence-based processes they need to acquire the knowledge and skills to engage with them in practice in the first place.

Definitions of EBP and EBN tend to refer to decision-making related to clinical interventions, although some read a little awkwardly. Melnyk and Fineout-Overholt's definition, for instance, refers to EBP as solving a problem whilst a number of nursing interventions are not problems, but either potential problems, or as indicated by Flemming (2008) interventions that are therapeutic, preventive, diagnostic or organisational. EBN can therefore be defined as holistic clinical interventions that are based on information that is available from valid and reliable relevant research, national clinical guidelines and expert healthcare professionals.

Hamer (2005: 6) suggests that the process of EBP is one that involves finding, appraising and applying scientific evidence to treatments in the management of health, the ultimate goal of which is to 'support practitioners in their decision-making in order to eliminate the use of ineffective, inappropriate, too expensive and potentially dangerous practices'.

There are several offshoots from the concept of EBP, such as EBN, evidence-based healthcare (EBHC) that (Gray, 2001) suggests is an approach to decision-making that entails the clinician using the 'best evidence' available; evidence-based medicine (EBM); evidence-based management; evidence-based education or teaching; and evidence-based assessment of healthcare profession students' clinical competencies. EBP refers to single clinical interventions (by a nurse/midwife/doctor/AHP), while EBHC tends to refer to groups of patients or health problems.

Thus, EBP involves making clinical intervention decisions based on the 'best evidence' that is currently available, which is appraised in the context of the professional experience of team members. The impact of the evidence is continually appraised thereafter. Following this brief overview of EBP, a more substantial examination of how practice teachers incorporate EBP in their day-to-day professional activities will be presented later in this chapter.

The reasons for practice being evidence-based

In addition to the reasons made explicit in the definitions of EBP, several other reasons can be identified. Healthcare students develop their knowledge of EBP very early on in their professional education programmes. Various researchers and pioneers have defined and researched this component as an activity that entails engaging in regular reflection before, during and after a clinical intervention regarding the basis for the evidence by which the activity was performed the way it was. Under the domain 'Evidence-based practice', the NMC (2008a: 57) also notes that all 'Registrants' must 'Further develop their evidence base for practice to support their own personal and professional development and to contribute to the development of others'.

You should be able to identify several reasons for EBP from your own and colleagues' professional experience, such as endeavouring to base nursing, or all clinical interventions on research, and utilising the knowledge and experience of senior colleagues. Several reasons for EBP have been identified over the years, including:

- It makes nursing and healthcare profession interventions much more scientific, through research-based care and treatment.
- Society seems to expect their health issues to be resolved by appropriately knowledgeable and educated experts.
- Managerialism and accountability – which refers to the notion that in the endeavour to achieve targets for healthcare set by the Department of Health (e.g. DH, 2009c), managers must be continuously inquisitive with regard to the rationales and efficiency of particular clinical interventions, i.e. whether the outcome can be achieved at a lower financial cost, and even whether the intervention should be performed at all.
- The quest for autonomy and professionalism – whereby each healthcare profession builds on its own core knowledge from research and learning from experience.
- Evidence-based practice as also a component of the clinical governance framework that incorporates clinical audits, risk management, patient-satisfaction monitoring and benchmarking, with all of these having implications for accountability.

Other reasons for EBP identified over the years by students on mentor courses include:

- The quest for the highest standards of care and treatment.
- All healthcare professionals performing clinical interventions to the same standard.
- Consistency across healthcare professionals through the use of the same evidence-based clinical guidelines and procedures.
- Comprising a standard that can be defended in case of litigation.
- Focusing on the effectiveness of clinical interventions.
- Providing a benchmark for ascertaining patient satisfaction with care and treatment.
- Ensuring practice is up to date.

Another reason for practice teachers ensuring their practice is evidence-based is that it is also one of the eight domains of knowledge and competence for practice teacher roles identified by the NMC (2008a: 57) for supporting learning and assessment in practice, the 'overall descriptor' for which is: 'Apply evidence-based practice to their own work and contribute to the further development of such a knowledge and practice evidence base'. The practice teacher outcomes for EBP are to:

- Identify areas of research and practice development based on an interpretation of existing evidence.
- Use local and national health frameworks to review and identify developmental needs.
- Advance their own knowledge and practice in order to develop new practitioners, at both registration levels and education at a level beyond initial registration, to be able to meet changes in practice roles and care delivery.
- Disseminate findings from research and practice development to enhance practice and the quality of learning experiences.

Another domain that is explored later in this chapter is 'Context of practice', which incorporates practice development and in turn explores informed change in methods of clinical interventions.

Sources, types and hierarchies of evidence

There are several sources of evidence on which clinical interventions can be based.

Action point 4.1 – Sources of evidence for specialist and advanced clinical practice

Identify and list all possible sources of evidence that you use, or could use, to inform clinical interventions in your clinical setting. This activity can be undertaken individually or in pairs.

Going by the definitions of EBP, the concept therefore focuses on the evidence by which clinicians will base their care and treatment, which can include research findings as well as the professional experiences of senior healthcare professionals. Box 4.1 identifies several other sources of evidence.

Box 4.1　Sources of evidence

- National clinical guidelines by, e.g., NICE
- Specialism specific healthcare journals
- Trust-based resource librarian
- Journals on EBP, e.g. evidence-based medicine

(Continued)

(Continued)

- Systematic reviews stored in e-databases, e.g. Cochrane library
- Specialist conference presentations
- ...

- Knowledge and experience of CNSs, ANPs, consultant nurses
- Senior doctors
- Benchmarking activities

The evidence available can be grouped as hierarchies of evidence, classifying these in groups from very strong evidence to more subjective evidence such as that based on professional expertise and experience. They can be classified as types or grades of evidence, and one such classification which is provided by Bandolier (2009) (a monthly journal addressing EBP) characterises EBP as types I to type IV, with the former referring to strong evidence from at least one systematic review of RCT, and the latter, at the other end of the spectrum, constituting personal experience by healthcare professionals. Bandolier's classification of evidence in EBP can be illustrated as a hierarchy – see Figure 4.1.

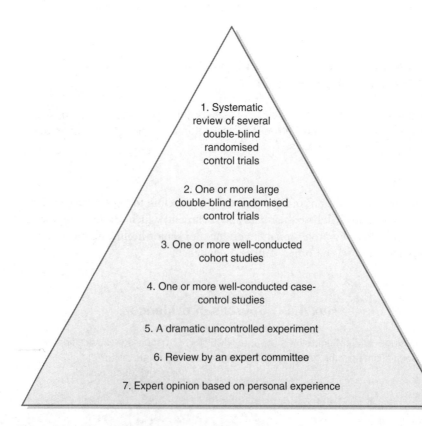

1. Systematic review of several double-blind randomised control trials

2. One or more large double-blind randomised control trials

3. One or more well-conducted cohort studies

4. One or more well-conducted case-control studies

5. A dramatic uncontrolled experiment

6. Review by an expert committee

7. Expert opinion based on personal experience

Figure 4.1   *Hierarchies of evidence in EBP*

Reviewing all relevant research on a particular item is referred to as a systematic review, which entails finding all relevant studies, published and unpublished, assessing each study, synthesising the findings from individual studies in an unbiased way and presenting a balanced and impartial summary of the findings with due consideration to any flaws in the evidence (Bandolier, 2009). Such systematic reviews usually provide a quantitative estimate of net benefit aggregated over all the studies included, which is an approach that is also termed meta-analysis.

The processes of systematic reviews comprise the following actions (Bandolier, 2009):

1 Defining an appropriate therapeutic question – i.e. a clear statement of the intervention of interest, relevant patient groups and the setting where the intervention is administered, as well as the appropriate outcomes.
2 Carefully searching all literature – including non-English sources, published and unpublished controlled trials of this intervention, studies reported at conferences and in company reports (including unpublished), plus those reported in non-leading journals, or unreported.
3 Assessing each study – for its eligibility for inclusion, the study quality and reported findings, preferably involving two independent reviewers.
4 Combining the findings from the individual studies – and aggregating them to produce a clear synthesis in quantitative terms.
5 Placing the findings in context – by aggregating the unbiased selection of studies and discussing them to address such issues as the quality and heterogeneity of the included studies, the likely impact of bias and chance, and the applicability of the findings.

Systematic reviews appear at the top of the hierarchy of evidence and other forms of evidence appear lower down in the hierarchy. An alternative and even more recent classification that identifies four levels of evidence to conclusions drawn in systematic reviews is provided by the Joanna Briggs Institute (JBI) (2008). The four levels of evidence in systematic reviews are further differentiated by the JBI in grades of recommendation for each component of evidence as to whether it also achieves feasibility, appropriateness, meaningfulness and effectiveness. The four levels of evidence for 'appropriateness' for instance are:

Level 1: metasynthesis of research with unequivocal synthesised findings
Level 2: metasynthesis of research with credible synthesised findings
Level 3: (a) metasynthesis of text/opinion with credible synthesised findings, and (b) one or more single research studies of high quality
Level 4: expert opinion.

Table 4.1 provides a summary of the three grades of recommendations from 'strongly supported' to 'not supported'.

Giving consideration to hierarchies of evidence will clearly assist healthcare professionals to make decisions on whether the evidence is sufficiently applicable and strong enough to base a clinical intervention on.

Clarke (1999) cites the use of 'gold standard' to describe and recommend the use of the best available evidence in clinical interventions. However, one of the

Table 4.1   *Grades of recommendations of EBP*

Grade of recommendations	Feasibility	Appropriateness	Meaningfulness	Effectiveness
Grade A	Strong support that merits application	Strong support that merits application	Strong support that merits application	Strong support that merits application
Grade B	Moderate support that warrants consideration of application	Moderate support that warrants consideration of application	Moderate support that warrants consideration of application	Moderate support that warrants consideration of application
Grade C	Not supported	Not supported	Not supported	Not supported

weaknesses of the term 'gold standard' is that although it may constitute the most suitable intervention for a particular condition, it may not suit everyone with that condition. This is because individuals react differently in terms of physiology to specific clinical interventions and the 'gold standard' intervention might be futile for particular individuals. Namely, what is 'gold standard' for one individual might not be so for another. Consequently, other clinical interventions which are of a lesser standard than 'gold' might be more suitable, but may not have been approved by the National Institute for Health and Clinical Excellence (NICE).

Satchell (2008) reports on a situation that identified the medication Sunitinib for advanced and/or metastatic kidney cancer, which could prolong life by a year but wasn't available under the NHS because it had not been assessed by NICE. This suggests that even when 'gold standard' medication does exist, it might not be available to NHS patients, and therefore deprives them of the 'gold standard' clinical intervention. However, following strong campaigning by individuals and stakeholder authorities (e.g. Cancer Research UK), NICE (2009) reassessed the situation, and approved the drug the following year, which is therefore now available under the NHS.

Morris and Maynard (2009) report on a study in which three third-year adult branch pre-registration nursing students and mentors participated in the implementation of EBP in a cardiac intensive care unit. They report that students demonstrated modest improvements in their knowledge and skills of EBP.

Action point 4.2 – Applying EBP to practice teaching

For the competence 'Apply evidence-based practice to their own work and contribute to the further development of such a knowledge and practice evidence base' under the domain 'evidence based practice' (NMC, 2008a: 57), explore how these practice teacher outcomes could be usefully applied to your area of work in the context of practice teaching and in specialist or advanced practice.

1 Identify areas of research and practice development based on an interpretation of existing evidence.
2 Use local and national health frameworks to review and identify developmental needs.

3 Advance own knowledge and practice in order to develop new practitioners, at both registration levels and education at a level beyond initial registration, and to be able to meet changes in practice roles and care delivery.
4 Disseminate findings from research and practice development to enhance practice and the quality of learning experiences.

Interpreting existing evidence for specialist and advanced clinical practice

One of the key components of EBP is appraising evidence prior to implementing its recommendations. This notion refers to appraising existing research related to a particular clinical intervention or health problem. Typically, appraising the evidence entails searching the literature for existing research on the specific intervention or problem, especially those based on RCTs. It is very important to note of course that other quantitative and qualitative studies can also be reviewed systematically.

RCTs tend to include research comparing two groups of subjects. In mental-health care, for instance, Embling (2002) reports on a study of cognitive behaviour therapy (CBT) that entailed the comparison of 19 clients who received 12 sessions of the treatment, with 19 clients as control group. They found that it is an effective treatment for depression, as also reported by Fava et al. (2004) amongst several others in their six-year comparative study that CBT is a more effective clinical intervention for recurrent depression than is clinical (i.e. medication-based) management.

The effectiveness of CBT for various conditions has also been systematically reviewed by the Cochrane Collaboration that identifies all research on the particular clinical intervention, critiques each study, draws conclusions from the exercise, and then makes recommendations. For this specific intervention the Cochrane Collaboration has systematically reviewed the effect of CBT on various health problems such as chronic pain management, adults with HIV, young sexual offenders, anxiety disorder and schizophrenia.

Thus systematic reviews and meta-analyses are performed on research on particular clinical interventions and stored in international databases such as the Cochrane Library; another prominent organisation that does this is the Joanna Briggs Institute. Health profession journals, for example the *Journal of Advanced Nursing*, report on recently conducted systematic reviews. Some will do this sporadically, others more regularly. For example, in January 2009, the *Journal of Advanced Nursing* published 'Review Summaries' (anon., 2009) on psychological therapies for generalised anxiety disorder; traction for low-back pain; water for wound cleansing, and embracing cultural diversity for developing and sustaining a healthy work environment in healthcare. For a systematic review of the use of water for wound cleansing, for instance, the review had been conducted by Fernandez et al. (2006) on behalf of the Joanna Briggs Institute. In this review the authors analysed nine trials (representing over 2500 participants) on the use of tap water to cleanse wounds, and concluded that there was insufficient evidence to either support or refute the use of tap water for wound cleansing.

A wide range of clinical interventions was reviewed such as children with type 1 diabetes, adults with generalised anxiety disorder, and so on. Some instances of clinical interventions reviewed by the Cochrane Collaboration (2009) are presented in Box 4.2.

Box 4.2   Instances of updated systematically reviewed clinical interventions by the Cochrane Collaboration (A of A to Z)

- Abdominal decompression for suspected fetal compromise/pre-eclampsia
- Acupuncture for migraine prophylaxis
- Admission avoidance and hospital at home
- Amantadine and rimantadine for influenza A in adults
- Antenatal perineal massage for reducing perineal trauma
- Antibiotic prophylaxis for operative vaginal delivery
- Antibiotics for acute bronchitis
- Antibiotics for spontaneous bacterial peritonitis in cirrhotic patients
- Antibiotics for treating acute chest syndrome in people with sickle cell disease
- Anticholinergic drugs for wheezing in children under the age of two years
- Anticoagulation for the long-term treatment of venous thromboembolism in patients with cancer
- Aromatherapy for dementia
- Aspirin or anticoagulants for treating recurrent miscarriage in women without antiphospholipid syndrome
- Assisted hatching on assisted conception (IVF and ICSI)
- Azathioprine or 6-mercaptopurine for the maintenance of remission in Crohn's disease

Source: Cochrane Collaboration (2009)

The Cochrane Library is only one of a few repositories of systematic reviews of clinical interventions available on the internet. Others include library databases such as MEDLINE and CINAHL through associated universities.

Cognitive behaviour therapy, that has above been referred to above, is an example of EBP that relevant specialist and advanced practitioners can implement in their areas of care and treatment. Other examples were noted in the preceding section. However, as indicated earlier in this chapter, systematically reviewed evidence is only one of many forms of evidence which specialist and advanced practitioners, and in fact all healthcare professionals, can base their care on. Where the method or the way in which the clinical intervention is conducted is changed to improve care delivery or the outcome for the patient or service user, this is referred to as practice development. This concept is one of the roles of the practice teacher, and is examined shortly in this chapter.

Issues related to EBP

Commentators on EBP strongly advise that RCTs should not be treated as the 'gold standard' evidence for all circumstances. This is because there are several other forms of evidence, and also because each individual, being different to some extent, might respond to the 'best evidence' intervention a little differently. Clinicians therefore must always give consideration to the application of evidence to the particular patient – different from EBHC that tends to consider evidence of clinical intervention related to groups of patients or to a particular health problem.

Thus, caution is advised against being so focused on evidence that the individualism of the patient is overlooked, as when a particular evidence is seen as the 'gold standard' intervention for a particular health problem. McKenna et al. (2004) argue that healthcare professionals are becoming more accountable within clinical governance structures for the care they provide, and therefore the need to use robust research findings effectively is a critical component of their role. However, as previous studies had shown, there are a number of potential obstacles that can hamper the effective use of best available evidence. McKenna et al. (2004) conducted a study to identify barriers to evidence-based practice in primary care, and found that many healthcare professionals wrongly believe that their practice is evidence based if to them EBP only means research based.

Sackett et al. (1996: 71) note that '. . . without available evidence, practice risks becoming rapidly out of date to the detriment of patients'. However, Bandolier (2009) warns that some of the published systematic reviews can be flawed due to inadequate reviewing expertise by the reviewer(s) or a lack of attention to detail, and also because not all systematic reviews are rigorous and unbiased.

Concerns related to securing consensus by all members of the team regarding appropriateness and timeliness of specific items of evidence prior to implementation require utilising the principles of management of change (discussed later in this chapter) every time EBP warrants making changes to practice.

Action point 4.3 – Barriers to developing and using EBP skills

Think about the scope of EBP in your role as practice teacher in your workplace, and identify the problematic areas in ascertaining that your practice is evidence-based on a day-to-day level.

The main barriers to developing EBP skills and implementing new evidence are a lack of time, the clinical setting's culture, difficulties in accessing on-line resources (Morris and Maynard, 2009; Palfreyman et al., 2003) and a lack of knowledge (Koehn and Lehman, 2008).

Furthermore, Kitson (2009) observes that there is a mismatch between the theories used to explain and influence clinical practice and the way in which the new knowledge is transferred into practice. She suggests that there is an implicit adherence to the view that healthcare systems operate totally mechanically in a logico–deductive fashion, and that successful innovation is a function of the level of local autonomy experienced by individuals and teams, and the involvement of key stakeholders.

In the above-cited study, McKenna et al. (2004) also found that the barriers cited by general practitioners were different from those cited by community nurses. While general practitioners believed that the most significant barriers to using evidence in practice included difficulty in keeping up with all the current changes in primary care and the ability to search for evidence-based information, those identified by community nurses were poor computer facilities, poor patient compliance and difficulties in influencing changes within primary care. McKenna et al. conclude that these two groups may require different strategies for barrier removal, which should consequently result in more efficient use of services.

The practice teacher as a practice developer

The role of the practice teacher encompasses practice development, and therefore this section explores our current understanding of various facets of the concept, and incorporates the notion of nurse entrepreneurs.

Current perspectives on clinical practice development

Making changes to procedures and protocols for clinical interventions, namely to the ways in which care and treatment are delivered, is not new, as this has been happening throughout the history of nursing and medicine in the endeavour to make clinical interventions more effective. Such changes, whenever they are based on research or experience, are referred to as practice development. The concept has proliferated in the last couple of decades to emphasise its significance in ensuring that methods of clinical interventions evolve and change as pertinent new evidence surfaces, thereby ensuring that clinical practice is 'informed'.

The NMC (2008a) identifies practice development as an activity that the practice teacher must be competent in. Under the domain 'context of practice', the overall descriptor states that the practice teacher must be able to 'Support learning within a context of practice that reflects healthcare and educational policies, managing change to ensure that particular professional needs are met within a learning environment that also supports practice development'. The practice teacher outcomes for 'context of practice' are:

- to recognise the unique needs of practice and contribute to the development of an environment that supports the achievement of NMC standards of proficiency
- to set and maintain professional boundaries, whilst at the same time recognising the contribution of the wider inter-professional team and the context of care delivery
- to support students in exploring new ways of working and the impact this may have on established professional roles.

The 'context of practice' domain, however, also incorporates input by the wider inter-professional team and new ways of working and their impact. Simultaneously, whilst enhancing their own practice and proficiency, the practice teacher also acts as a role model to others to enable them to learn safe and effective clinical interventions.

Various definitions of practice development have been presented over time. McSherry and Warr (2008), for example, identified several definitions presented between 1994 and 2006. (Other definitions are likely to have been synthesised since 2006.) Essentially, based on the extant knowledge on practice development, it can be defined as minor, substantial or major changes that are made to the process or methods of clinical interventions that are based on current knowledge in the profession that aspires to deliver the safest and most effective practice.

McCormack (2009: 160–1) elaborates that 'practice development is a systematic and rigorous approach to working collaboratively and inclusively with clinicians and service users using participatory and critical engagement in the transformation of the social, cultural, discursive and material conditions of practice, to bring about person-centred cultures'. McCormack (2009) also identifies the principles that underpin all practice development work as collaboration, inclusion and participation.

Practice development is supported by various policy publications, for example the CNO's identification of ten key roles for nurses that were initially incorporated in *The NHS Plan* (DH, 2000) (as identified in Chapter 1, Box 1.3) and in (DH 2002) *Developing Key Roles for Nurses and Midwives – A Guide for Managers*, and it forms part of the *NHS KSF* (DH, 2004a) under the 'core' dimensions of service improvement and quality in particular, as well as the general dimension of 'development and innovation'.

Instances of practice development

Practice development is by no means a new phenomenon, as ways in which patient and service-user care is delivered and techniques of clinical interventions, many of which are subsequently incorporated into procedures and clinical guidelines, have been changing throughout the history of nursing and healthcare. In learning support roles, more than two decades ago, Darling's (1984) research into the characteristics and roles of mentors identified the activities and qualities as being a role model, an envisioner, and a standard-prodder as components that constitute practice development.

Further examples of practice development (akin to service improvement) cited in healthcare literature include a wide range of novel clinical activities such as new nurse-led clinics, and in acute-care areas, rapid tranquilisation for the management of agitated patients (Care Services Improvement Partnership, 2009).

Changes that improve care and treatment are generally supported by the government, such as can be seen in their White Paper *Our Health, Our Care, Our Say* (DH, 2006b), which cites various case studies as instances of practice development in primary-care services, for example:

- Improving mental health in London – pioneering work in mental health, including work with local voluntary and community services and the use of employment advisers to enable people to go back to work, and remain in employment.
- Pharmacy-based anti-coagulant monitoring gives instant results in Durham – pharmacies are offering innovative new services that could improve compliance, as some patients choose not to go to the hospital for monitoring because it is inconvenient or decide not to take their anti-coagulant anymore.
- Self-testing available on the high street in London for sexually transmitted diseases – encouraging young adults to test themselves for STIs, through a partnership

between Boots and the Department of Health (as young people do not always use traditional health services, but most tend to buy beauty products) has led to chlamydia-screening kits being available in Boots stores across the capital.

- Nurses near you in Blackburn – a district nursing team helped to set up a mobile clinic for men, especially those from ethnic minorities, many of whom do not speak English.
- Nurse-practitioner-led outreach services in Huddersfield – focusing on a particularly deprived area, the service supports nearly 17,000 families with children, providing immunisation and vaccinations, contraception and advice on sexual health, teenage-pregnancy clinics, child-health surveillance and help with smoking cessation.

Furthermore, in *Our Health, Our Care, Our Say – One Year On*, the Department of Health (2007d) cites several priorities for the 12 months following, including:

- better access to psychological therapies and crisis support
- end-of-life care networks in place in every area
- single assessment/care plan for those with ongoing needs
- using new technology to help people live independently
- new bowel cancer screening
- promoting understanding of mental wellbeing
- Fitter Britain campaign.

The process of practice development

The practice teacher is therefore required to have an enquiring mind, and to be alert and constantly pursuing the quest for better ways of working, which will benefit patients' and service users' health and wellbeing. They can therefore explore development in all components of their role, namely those identified by the Scottish government for instance (2008), which are clinical practice, leadership and organisation of care, patient education and research. The RCN provides guidelines and support for nurses engaging in projects on practice development.

The process of practice development comprises identifying specific areas of patient healthcare needs for which either new practice or changes to practice are required. For example, if a need is identified for an improved method for treating leg ulcers, or for dealing with substance abuse in a particular locality, then healthcare professionals can explore this and make changes in a planned and systematic way. The change has to be managed systematically, and ways of doing so are explored later in this chapter.

Nurse entrepreneurs

The practice teacher's role includes leadership, which in Mintzberg's (1990) study of management roles is also identified as 'entrepreneurial roles', which in turn implies implementing novel, usually unprecedented concepts, namely innovating. Entrepreneurship therefore overlaps to some extent with the concepts of clinical-practice development and the management of change (discussed later). It is a relatively recent and still unfolding concept that is supported by government policy (DH, 2008b) as 'social enterprise'.

With regards to nurse entrepreneurship, Drennan et al. (2007) conducted an integrative literature review of entrepreneurial nurses and midwives in the UK to investigate the extent of entrepreneurial activity by nurses and midwives, and the factors that influenced these activities. They reported that nurse entrepreneurship is an under-researched area, and that the number of nurses, midwives and SCPHNs acting entrepreneurially in the UK and internationally was very small. They categorised entrepreneurial activity by employment status and product and constructed a typology of entrepreneurs:

1   Employees as entrepreneurs (referred to as intrapreneurs), who focused on innovations and changes pioneered as part of their job role.
2   Those providing services indirectly related to healthcare, such as nurse consultancies, infrastructure and workforce providers, and inventors/manufacturers.
3   Employees or self-employed healthcare professionals providing other direct healthcare services, including complementary therapists, and nurse-general practitioner partners.
4   Entrepreneurial decisions in care and residential homes.

They concluded that nurse entrepreneurship involves venturesome individuals who stimulate economic progress by developing new ways of doing things, and can exploit opportunities and mobilise resources. They also observed that the extent to which nurses and midwives respond to calls for greater entrepreneurialism is also influenced by the complex interplay of contextual factors (e.g. healthcare legislation), professional and managerial experience, and demographic factors.

Entrepreneurship in nursing is not necessarily nurse focused in that as innovators they provide a service where there has been a previous gap in healthcare provision. As noted earlier, various instances of nurse entrepreneurship are publicised in Department of Health documents (e.g. DH, 2006b). The Royal College of Nursing (2007b) document *Nurse Entrepreneurs – Turning Initiative into Independence* provides further guidelines and support for entrepreneurial nurses. The ICN (2004) also provides guidelines for nurse entrepreneurs and intrapreneurs and discusses their prevalence, their roles, the services they provide, and their profiles in terms of personal qualities and qualifications.

Mooney (2009a) reports on instances of nurse entrepreneurship that entail nurse-led general practices that involve the nurse employing their own general medical practitioners as well. However, ultimately, the prime focus of nurse entrepreneurship is to initiate new nursing interventions that will benefit patients and service users.

The practice teacher as 'researcher'

As identified for several years now, the nurse's role includes a knowledge of research in nursing and healthcare, and even more so in the practice teacher's role as a specialist or advanced practitioner. Some practice-based nurses conduct research or are part of a team of researchers on specific projects. At times practice development forms the basis for research in that the change in the clinical intervention method is scientifically evaluated, or it is explored using the action-research method.

The term research has different interpretations depending on the context in which it is being deliberated. It can refer to well-designed scientific studies, or to applied research, which refers to several forms of searching for knowledge.

However, the majority of nurses will only go as far as having a knowledge of the mechanics of, and on the look out for, new research findings in their specialism or area of practice, and this coincides with various examples of barriers to the implementation of research findings that have been documented over the years (e.g. McKenna et al., 2004; Kitson, 2009). Comino and Kemp (2008) reported on a study that explored research-related activities in community-based child-health services, and concluded that an increased focus on EBP has created expectations that community-based child-health-service staff could utilise, and could also contribute to research evidence. They indicated that whilst there is interest among community-based child-health-service staff in participating in research related activities, an investment in leadership, skills development, infrastructure, resources and novel ways to enhance research output within these services is needed to increase participation.

Practice teachers also need to ensure that they have developed skills in critical appraisal or critiquing published research. For this reason they should be able to evaluate how valid and reliable the studies they are interested in are. Guidelines on how to critique individual research studies abound in the literature (e.g. Lipp, 2007; Gopee, 2008a). Guidelines for systematic reviews are also presented in various publications – see Box 4.3.

Box 4.3   Guidelines for systematic reviews

- Is the topic well defined?
- Was the search for papers thorough?
- Were criteria for the inclusion of studies clearly described and fairly applied?
- Was study quality assessed by blinded or independent reviewers?
- Was missing information sought from the original study investigators?
- Do the included studies seem to indicate similar effects?
- Were the overall findings assessed for their robustness?
- Was the play of chance assessed?
- Are the recommendations based firmly on the quality of the evidence presented?

Source: Bandolier, 2009

Furthermore, Bandolier (2009) warns that not all systematic reviews are rigorous and unbiased, and provides a set of questions as a framework for interrogating individual systematic reviews. Nonetheless, substantial systematic reviews have already been performed for clinicians by organisations such as the Cochrane Collaboration, and specific examples of systematically appraised research on clinical interventions related to specialist and advanced practice can also be accessed through their website (see References for examples).

However, systematic reviews can of course be performed by individual practitioners, which can be lodged on the Cochrane Collaboration Library if the latter's guidelines are strictly adhered to. For example, McGaughey et al. (2007) systematically reviewed the utilisation of outreach and early warning systems (EWS) for the prevention of intensive care admission and the death of critically ill adult patients on general hospital wards (available from the Cochrane Library website), and found that EWS led to a reduction in hospital mortality compared with the control group. The authors, however, expressed concern about the poor methodological quality of most of the studies.

Disseminating findings from research and innovative clinical practices

There are, of course, numerous research studies on the effectiveness of specialist and advanced practice roles in relation to how far their clinical interventions benefit patients and service users, that is in terms of patient outcomes (e.g. Maughan and Clarke, 2001; Fava et al., 2004). How do healthcare professionals get to know about the findings of these studies and innovative clinical practices? Dissemination of findings from research and practice development to enhance practice is one of the roles and areas of competence of the practice teacher (NMC, 2008a).

Hundley et al. (2000) reported on a project that was designed to raise research awareness among midwives and nurses, which resulted in a significant increase in both knowledge and the use of research resources. Le May et al. (1998) explored research cultures, and found that many factors, both individual and organisational, affect research utilisation, and that practitioners and managers hold differing perceptions of the nature and role of research, and the opportunities and constraints which affect its dissemination and utilisation.

Action point 4.4 – Dissemination of findings from research and practice development

Based on your (own) experience and knowledge, jot down a number of ways in which findings from research and innovative clinical practices are disseminated by healthcare professionals, in both your workplace, and nationally and internationally, in addition to the ways in which researchers and practice developers do so.

Researchers and practice developers disseminate their findings by making their research theses available in academic libraries, by publication of the study as journal articles or monographs, and by conference presentations. Other media for disseminating research findings include less formal means, such as staff meetings, informal work-related conversations, local presentations and drawing attention to research encountered on study days and courses, and even through computer networks such as Facebook, and on-line learning discussions. As a competent leader, the practice teacher is expected to apply existing and new evidence-based knowledge to clinical practice and to engage fully with change implementation (NMC, 2008a). New ways of working can be introduced, imposed or managed.

New ways of working and their impact

Practice development and EBP both comprise changing practice as and when new modes of clinical interventions are advocated from research and innovation pilot study projects. These new ways of working are more effectively implemented if the principles of change management are operationalised.

Changes in practice roles and care delivery

Why are there changes in healthcare? There are various reasons for such changes occurring in healthcare delivery. Changes are generally made to the way care is delivered when research or an evaluation highlights problems or more effective ways of providing care, or when complaints have been received. At other times they are made due to new policy decisions and directives; or when individual healthcare professionals trial and prove other ways of performing clinical interventions or care provisions that can lead to better patient outcomes.

Managing innovation and change

Leadership is a key attribute of the dual teacher-cum-specialist or advanced practitioner roles. When a change in clinical activity is required, whether it is related to a change in clinical practice, the organisation of care or in teaching students or patients, that change is best implemented through a systematic management of change approach to ensure its effectiveness. What are the ways in which change can be managed effectively? The literature cites various frameworks or models that can be utilised for the systematic management of change in professional clinical practice.

Managing change entails planning how that change will be implemented, and when and which pre-conditions need to be in place, such as adequate resources. There are several guidelines in the literature on how to manage change. For example, having noted that the knowledge transfer from research to clinical settings is a slow and haphazard process, Graham et al. (2006: 13) suggested a conceptual framework that can enable 'knowledge creation and knowledge application'. The framework comprises commonly identified steps in the management of change. Such steps are also captured by Gopee and Galloway (2009) in their systematic framework for managing change using the 'seven-step RAPSIES model for effective change management'. It is presented diagrammatically in Figure 4.2, and Box 4.4 provides brief details of each component of the RAPSIES model.

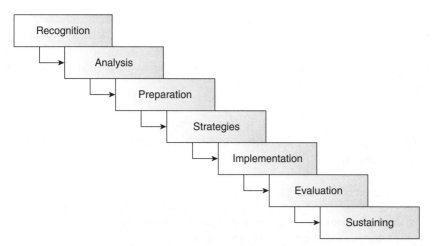

Figure 4.2   *The seven-step RAPSIES framework for managing change effectively*

Box 4.4   Details of the RAPSIES framework for managing change effectively

The seven-step model comprises the essential components of the management of change, which are as follows:

1 **Recognising** the need to improve an element of practice or for change to solve a problem for instance.
2 **Analysing** the available options related to the contemplated change, such as the setting in which the change will be implemented and the users of that change.
3 **Preparing** for the change, such as identifying a change agent who will lead the implementation of the change and the education required, defining the intended outcomes and involving the relevant individuals.
4 **Strategies** that are chosen for implementing the change.
5 **Implementing** the change, including the piloting and timing of this implementation.
6 **Evaluating** the effectiveness of the change against the intended outcomes.
7 **Sustaining** the change to ensure that it endures and is mainstreamed.

Source: Gopee and Galloway, 2009

The RAPSIES model should prove an effective framework for managing change in nursing interventions as it is synthesised from extant literature and research published over several years. In implementing this framework, either the initiator of the change or the change agent should feel at liberty to modify or adapt the components or steps of the model so that it is tuned to the local setting's values and culture, and can thereby enhance the likelihood of an effective implementation. It is also useful to note that although it is suggested that a sequential approach to managing change will be appropriate, the initiator or change agent should be aware that the sequencing of the model should not be treated as rigid linear uni-directional steps that have to be adhered to, and therefore it can be viewed as a spiral in which certain steps or components can be revisited or, if required, reworked before progressing on to the next step.

> ## Action point 4.5 – Further considerations in implementing new evidence
>
> Barriers to implementing research and EBP were considered earlier in this chapter. Other than barriers to change, and looking again at the RAPSIES model, what do you feel are any other factors that need to be considered by, say, the change agent to ensure a successful implementation?

Certain steps, for example '*Preparation*' for the change, may need to be worked in assimmilable chunks, and therefore some educational preparation of the users of the change may need to occur at the beginning of the venture, with the rest a short while later, and so on. Another example is in relation to a '*Recognition*' of the need for change in that the users of the change may not recognise the need, nor be ready for the change until they have sufficient educational preparation, which in this model is identified as the third step.

Change implementation might require specific extra resources, which the change agent will need to identify as precisely as they can. This could signify extra funds for additional staffing, and/or for the purchase of equipment, devices or consumables (i.e. disposable materials). He or she will need to take into account who to negotiate the extra resources with. They may need to consider who has the power to make decisions for approving extra funds. Political strategies such as persuading influential allies might also play a key role in the acquisition of other resources.

Another factor that needs to be considered is the actions that can be taken should they encounter problems at any stage of the RAPSIES framework, or with any of the other factors just identified, or if the implementation appears to be failing. Therefore, details of the factors that will be required to 'sustain' the change are, of course, also crucial. Another problematic eventuality to be prepared for is in case the change agent him or herself is subject to other calls. For instance, if the change agent is a modern matron leading a change to avert a risk, or is a CNS, then on occasion he or she might be asked to undertake other clinical activities, such as to manage a unit for a few shifts in times of staffing crises, or during an epidemic, if such a provision is built into the post role.

Mockett et al. (2006) explored education leadership (which is discussed further in Chapter 7) in the practice setting with regard to a new framework for clinical nursing education that was introduced in a part of New Zealand in response to the significant legislative and post-registration nursing education changes. Building on the existing published literature on the management of change, they developed a four-stage approach to implementing the framework, which comprised:

Stage 1: the identification process of the impetus for change.

Stage 2: creating a realistic and sustainable vision of what the change would look like within the organisation, so as to ensure success, and to guide the process of change.

Stage 3: implementing the vision and discussing the communication and pilot phase of implementation.

Stage 4: exploring the process and experiences of changing the local culture and embedding the vision into an organisation.

Mockett et al. (2006) conclude by reinforcing the importance of implementing robust, consistent, strategic and collaborative processes – that reflect and evaluate best educational nursing practice – and that the journey of change requires clear management, strong leadership, perseverance and an understanding of an organisation's culture.

With regard to establishing and sustaining change in the context of evidence-based practice, Rycroft-Malone (2009) reports on a study that explored how magnet hospitals in the USA and non-magnet hospitals approach EBP. She reports that in magnet hospitals EBP is a norm, and a spontaneous and natural activity, whilst in non-magnet hospitals it has more superficial ownership.

Evaluating the effectiveness of practice development

As identified in stage six of the RAPSIES framework, a key component of the management of change is an evaluation of its intended effects after it has been implemented. An evaluation needs to be conducted formatively and summatively, and decisions should be made on actions that must be taken if weaknesses or problems are detected. This principle applies to practice development as well. The principles of evaluation are explored in detail in Chapter 7 as part of the leadership component of the practice teacher's role.

Conclusion

Chapter 4 examined the practice teacher's role in EBP in the context of specialist and advanced practice, and in practice development. Practice teachers as innovators and 'nurse entrepreneurs' are inherent concepts and activities that incorporate managing change and innovation, disseminating innovative clinical practices, and the practice teacher as 'researcher'. This chapter therefore addressed the following inherent components:

- The practice teacher as an evidence-based practitioner, and included definitions and a brief overview of EBP, identifying the reasons, sources and hierarchies of EBP, EBP in specialist and advanced clinical practice, and issues related to EBP.
- The practice teacher's role as practice developer, including current perspectives on practice development, and instances and processes of practice development and nurse entrepreneurship.
- The practice teacher as 'researcher', systematic review skills, and disseminating the findings from research and innovative clinical practices.
- New ways of working, that is managing change and innovations, and evaluating the effectiveness of practice development.

All registrants increasingly need to firm up their approach to their clinical activities as evidence-based practitioners, and in the light of new evidence and health-service needs, continue to develop their practice. Following on from this area of practice teacher competence, the focus of Chapter 5 will be on the assessment of knowledge and the competence of healthcare practitioners on specialist and advanced practice courses.

5

Assessing Specialist and Advanced Practice Knowledge and Competence

Introduction

Various dimensions of the practice teaching role were examined in the preceding chapters of this book. Chapter 5 focuses on the nature of assessments in healthcare education programmes, that is the definitions, reasons and methods of assessments, and the assessment of student knowledge and competence in pre-registration and in specialist and advanced practice programmes.

Chapter outcomes

On completion of this chapter you should be able to:

1   Critically evaluate the contemporary nature and principles of assessment of knowledge and competence in healthcare profession pre-registration and post-qualifying programmes, taking into account the general reasons for assessments, identifying levels of learning, assessment strategies, research, and patients' and service users' involvement in the assessment of competencies.
2   Demonstrate a critical understanding of ways of assessing how pre-registration education students perform essential skills safely and effectively, the evidence-base for deciding on pass or fail decisions, for confirming that students have or have not achieved their practice competencies, and the principles of giving feedback after assessments.
3   Critically analyse ways of assessing safe and effective specialist and advanced practice knowledge and the competence of students on specialist and advanced practice programmes, including cross-professional assessment.
4   Ascertain analytically how academic and professional standards related to healthcare education programmes are maintained in the context of national guidelines and standards.

The general nature of assessments – an overview

The assessment of specialist and advanced practice knowledge, competence and proficiencies is the most important function that the practice teacher has to fulfil. The first section of this chapter presents an analytical overview of what are assessments, and precisely what practice teachers assess, why and how.

Contemporary nature of assessments

An assessment of knowledge and competence can be understood by asking the general questions related to what assessments are, why they are performed and how assessments are performed, as well as considering research and healthcare professionals' day-to-day experiences of assessments.

Action point 5.1 – Assessments in practice

Think of all your experiences of assessment of both clinical skills (in clinical settings or clinical skills laboratories) and professional knowledge over the years, both as a student and as an assessor, and identify your personal thoughts on the reasons for assessments, and on the way they are conducted. Spend a few minutes on this, and make some notes.

In healthcare profession programmes students are assessed both on their clinical skills and their theoretical knowledge. There are occasions when there are issues, or even problems with assessments, for which there are usually established protocols that the assessor can follow.

What are assessments?

Practice teachers are experienced healthcare professionals who already have substantial knowledge of assessments, which they have developed predominantly from attending mentor preparation programmes and updates. Therefore the reader is expected to know specifically what is assessed on professional courses and how, and the general profession-specific reasons for conducting these assessments. Furthermore, they build on their existing knowledge and competence of assessments that healthcare professionals as practice teachers have.

In the context of an assessment of healthcare professionals' knowledge and competence, assessment refers to collecting and interpreting evidence of learning and competence presented by the student, and making decisions on the appropriateness and quality of the evidence against pre-determined criteria. Accordingly, Curzon (2003) indicates that assessments involve collecting, measuring and interpreting information relating to students' responses to the teaching they have received.

These definitions highlight assessment as a key component of learning. They incorporate ascertaining the quality, quantity and appropriateness of learning, and therefore the student's attainment and progress. They also clearly involve judging the merit of the evidence presented by a student on how far they meet the pre-set criteria, and then giving feedback to them so that they can learn further and build on the experience.

There are a number of essential dimensions of assessments that need careful consideration when incorporating methods of assessment within healthcare courses' curricula. These include:

- Which course and which module learning outcomes each component of assessment assesses – this also addresses the validity of the assessment component.
- Assessment parity – i.e. the extent of the demands the assessment makes on the student must be roughly equal across all modules at specific academic levels.
- The marking criteria used for awarding pass/fail or different bands of marks (usually from 0 per cent to 100 per cent). Some are graded, i.e. awarded grades between A and F.
- The pass mark – this can vary from 35 per cent for some coursework to 100 per cent (e.g. for the drug calculation component) for other kinds.
- Mechanisms for marking, internal moderation, external examining, and ratification of results at Examinations and Assessment Board meetings.

Assessing theoretical knowledge in health profession programmes

There are two principal strands of assessments in healthcare professional education programmes, which are (i) the assessment of theoretical knowledge, and (ii) the assessment of competencies (incorporates skills and practical knowledge), as also distinguished by Benner (2001). More fully, they assess students' demonstration of critically evaluated knowledge of the subject area, and then marks are awarded for comprehension, application, analysis, synthesis and the evaluation of designated topic areas, or coursework questions. These six components regarding assessment of theoretical work are based on Bloom's (1956) taxonomy of learning objectives (see Figure 5.1). Therefore, for lower levels, such as the first year of an undergraduate programme, students are awarded marks for evidence of learning at all taxonomy levels; and for the third year of the programme or higher levels, more marks are awarded for higher academic levels (analysis, synthesis and evaluation), and less for lower academic levels (knowledge and comprehension).

Bloom's taxonomy was not based on research but on the experience of education administrators (Biggs and Tang, 2007). More recently, after further work on Bloom's taxonomy, Anderson and Krathwohl (2001) developed a taxonomy for learning, teaching, and assessing, as presented in Figure 5.1.

Implementation of Anderson and Krathwohl's (2001) revised taxonomy should prove a very useful framework for planning education programmes, designing learning outcomes and teaching that matches students' levels of learning in nurse education. Biggs and Tang (2007) present a more recent research-based alternative taxonomy of learning referred to as SOLO (Structure of the Observed Learning Outcome):

Unistructural: memorising and recalling, recognising and ordering.
Multistructural: classifying, discussing, illustrating.
Relational: applying, analysing, explaining, problem-solving.
Extended abstract: theorising, generalising, hypothesising, creating.

Other frameworks for assessing theoretical knowledge are also available, which educational institutions can utilise. The QAA (2008b), for instance, presents

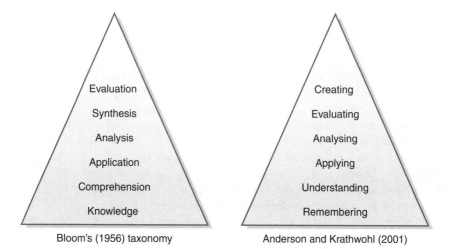

| Bloom's (1956) taxonomy | Anderson and Krathwohl (2001) |

Figure 5.1   *Taxonomy of learning*

Sources: Bloom, 1956; Anderson and Krathwohl, 2001

descriptors for learning at different academic levels, such as year one, two and three of the customary three-year undergraduate university course, but on a 1 to 9 scale for learning from very early stages to doctorate level. Box 5.1 illustrates the standard of preparation that is consistent with studying at degree level. QAA descriptors therefore form a guide for programme planning in university education.

Box 5.1   Descriptor for a higher education qualification at level 6: Bachelor's degree with honours

The descriptor provided for this level of the FHEQ is for any Bachelor's degree with honours which should meet the descriptor in full. This qualification descriptor can also be used as a reference point for other level 6 qualifications, including Bachelor's degrees, graduate diplomas, etc.

Bachelor's degrees with honours are awarded to students who have demonstrated:

- a systematic understanding of key aspects of their field of study, including the acquisition of coherent and detailed knowledge, at least some of which is at, or informed by, the forefront of defined aspects of a discipline
- an ability to deploy accurately established techniques of analysis and enquiry within a discipline
- conceptual understanding that enables the student:

  o to devise and sustain arguments, and/or to solve problems, using ideas and techniques, some of which are at the forefront of a discipline
  o to describe and comment upon particular aspects of current research, or equivalent advanced scholarship, in the discipline as an appreciation of the uncertainty, ambiguity and limits of knowledge

o the ability to manage their own learning and to make use of scholarly reviews and primary sources (for example, refereed research articles and/or original materials appropriate to the discipline).

Typically, holders of the qualification will be able to:
- apply the methods and techniques that they have learned to review, consolidate, extend and apply their knowledge and understanding, and to initiate and carry out projects
- critically evaluate arguments, assumptions, abstract concepts and data (that may be incomplete), to make judgements, and to frame appropriate questions to achieve a solution – or identify a range of solutions – to a problem
- communicate information, ideas, problems and solutions to both specialist and non-specialist audiences.

And holders will have:
- the qualities and transferable skills necessary for employment requiring:

  o the exercise of initiative and personal responsibility
  o decision-making in complex and unpredictable contexts
  o the learning ability needed to undertake appropriate further training of a professional or equivalent nature.

Source: QAA, 2008b

Assessing professional competencies at different levels

As with categorising levels of theoretical knowledge, levels of clinical practice can also be determined systematically by using research based frameworks such as those published by Steinaker and Bell (1979), Benner (2001), Bondy (1983) and Price (2008) (see Box 5.2).

Box 5.2   Frameworks for assessing professional practice at different levels

Level	Steinaker and Bell's (1979)	Benner's (2001)	Bondy's (1983)	Price's (2008)
1	Exposure	Novice	Dependent	Fundamental skills
2	Participation	Advanced beginner	Marginal	Intermediate skills
3	Identification	Competent	Assisted	Advanced skills
4	Internalisation	Proficient	Supervised	Sophisticated skills
5	Dissemination	Expert	Independent	

Price's (2008) skills taxonomy therefore identifies fundamental level skills, that is easier to learn skills, as at level 1, intermediate skills (the next higher level) as level 2, advanced skills as level 3, and highest level skills or 'sophisticated' skills as level 4. These levels can be incorporated in educational programmes to determine the level of skills that students are expected to learn during years 1, 2 and 3 of a three-year undergraduate university course (e.g. level 1 in year 1).

Achieving full 'mastery' of certain clinical skills can potentially take a relatively short period of time, but usually this can take several weeks, months or years. It also depends on how skills are defined. The term competence is generally used to signify the practical psychomotor dexterity required to perform the skill, but depending on alternative definitions, it can also signify incorporating practical knowledge and theoretical knowledge, as discussed in Chapter 8.

Why assess?

Taken from a broad general stance, it is possible to identify the general aims of assessments.

Action point 5.2: Aims of assessments

Remind yourself of the general aims of assessments, and of those that are specific for healthcare profession courses. Then consider specifically what the aims of assessment of students on specialist or advanced practice programmes are.

Details of the aims of assessments in healthcare courses have been pretty well documented (e.g. Quinn and Hughes, 2007; Gopee, 2008a), and generally constitute:

- to ascertain how competently the supervisee can perform specified clinical interventions
- to decide on the learner's 'fitness for practice' of the skill
- to record progress with the achievement of standards of proficiency/course outcomes
- to identify subsequent learning needs.

The aims of assessment apply to the practice teacher's assessment role as well, and include establishing 'fitness for purpose' and 'fitness for award' at specialist and advanced level practice. For the practice teacher, this means assessing the achievement of the identified professional competencies and the university's course requirements, that is practice outcomes. Fundamentally, the reason for assessing healthcare profession students' competencies is to ascertain if they value, and are capable of, 'safe and effective practice' (NMC, 2004b, 2008a).

The NMC (2008a) identifies the outcomes for practice teachers for the domain 'Assessment and accountability' as follows:

1 Set effective professional boundaries whilst creating a dynamic and constructive teacher-student relationship.
2 In partnership with other members of the teaching team, use knowledge and experience to design and implement assessment frameworks.
3 Be able to assess practice for registration, and also at a level beyond that of initial registration.
4 Provide constructive feedback to students and help them identify future learning needs and actions. Manage failing students so that they may either enhance their performance and capabilities for safe and effective practice, or be able to understand their failure and the implications of this for their future.
5 Be accountable for confirming that students have met, or not met, the NMC standards of proficiency in practice for registration – and at a level beyond initial registration – and are capable of safe and effective practice.

The concepts inherent in these outcomes are as follows. The first outcome suggests that for students to develop competence, a working teacher–student relationship is essential. This concept was explored in detail in Chapter 2. The second outcome emphasises the significance of healthcare professionals as members of a teaching team, that is a team that supports learning and assessment in the practice setting. The teaching team's remit includes agreeing on the means that will be utilised for assessing students' competencies.

The third outcome in this domain indicates that the practice teacher must be competent in assessing students' competencies for students on pre-registration preparation programme, as well as post-qualifying.

The fourth outcome addresses a number of components. First, it indicates that the practice teacher should be competent in providing feedback to the student after assessing them, and that this feedback needs to be consistent with best practice principles – this will be addressed later in this chapter. This outcome also recognises that some students may be under-achieving, that is failing to develop the competencies they are expected to achieve, and likely to have agreed to achieve in a learning contract by a particular stage in their professional education programme. The outcome indicates that the situation should be managed, implying that the practice teacher must be cognisant of this situation, and should ascertain exactly how the student is progressing with achieving these competencies. If this appears difficult or unachievable, then the practice teacher should inform and consult the specialist area's PEF or the link teacher.

This outcome goes even further, and indicates that the practice teacher should discuss the implications of the student's failure to achieve, both for patients' or service users' health and wellbeing, and for their own career.

Assessment strategies and frameworks

A number of well-known methods and strategies for the assessment of competence are available to practice teachers for an assessment of students' professional knowledge and competence, many of which are identified in Box 5.3.

Box 5.3   Strategies for assessing theory and practice

Strategies for assessing theory (i.e. theoretical knowledge)	Strategies for assessing practice (i.e. practical knowledge and competence)
• Seminars • Essays • Posters • Course portfolio • Reflective accounts • Concept maps • Multiple-choice questions • Work products	• Objective structured clinical examinations (OSCE) • Practice grid objectives • Work products • Reflective accounts/profile • Questioning • Simulations, to assess more senior students • Skill demonstration

More specifically, the areas to be assessed comprise all or specified module learning outcomes, which can be assessed through written assignments (assessing theoretical knowledge), and/or practice components through planned assessment of the NMC's (2004b) *Standards of Proficiency for Pre-registration Nurse Education.* The standards are translated into specific skills that are predominantly assessed during practice placements. The HPC has also published standards of proficiency for different allied health professions. Furthermore, for learning beyond initial registration, post-qualifying course competencies, and specialist or advanced practice competencies are also available.

The NMC (2004b) standards of proficiency for pre-registration nurse education are identified under four domains: professional and ethical practice, care delivery, care management, and personal and professional development. Under each domain, specific outcomes are identified for both the common foundation programme (CFP), and for the branch programmes separately. The outcomes for one component under the domain 'care delivery' are reproduced in Box 5.4.

Box 5.4   Domain, outcomes and standards for one component of the NMC's domain 'care delivery'

Domain	Outcomes to be achieved for entry to the branch programme	Standards of proficiency for entry to the register: care delivery
Care delivery *Contribute to the planning of nursing care, involving patients and clients and, where possible,*	• identify care needs based on the assessment of a patient or client • participate in the negotiation and agreement of the care plan with the patient or client and with their	• establish priorities for care based on individual or group needs • develop and document a care plan to achieve optimal health, habilitation, and

their carers; demonstrating an understanding of helping patients and clients to make informed decisions	carer, family or friends, as appropriate, under the supervision of a registered nurse • inform patients and clients about intended nursing actions, respecting their right to participate in decisions about their care	rehabilitation based on assessment and current nursing knowledge • identify expected outcomes, including a time frame for achievement and/or review in consultation with patients, clients, their carers and family and friends and with members of the health and social care team

The practice teacher's role incorporates an assessment of the competencies of pre-registration students at the signing-off proficiency stage of their programme. The specialist and advanced practice competencies or outcomes that students have to achieve have been constituted by various organizations (as noted in Chapter 1 and earlier in this chapter), including the NMC (2006a), the RCN (2008), the DH (2004a), the Scottish government (2008), the ICN (2001), *The National Education and Competence Framework for Advanced Critical Care Practitioners* (DH, 2008e) and by research (e.g. Gardner et al., 2007).

The latest generic outcomes for the specialist and advanced practice programme proffered by the NMC (2008b) are still under review. Those for SCPHNs identify the domains (DH, 2004a), principles and standards that SCPHN students need to achieve, that is to be assessed and deemed competent in to be able to register their qualification on the NMC register of specialist practitioners. The four domains are:

1 Search for health needs.
2 Stimulation of awareness of health needs.
3 Influence on policies affecting health.
4 Facilitation of health-enhancing activities.

The principles and standards for the first domain are presented in Table 3.1 in Chapter 3. However, some assessment components can address both theoretical knowledge and practical aspects as in assessed reflective accounts, and student-seminar presentations.

Assessment frameworks

Various methods and strategies for assessing students have been identified over time including those for assessing students on healthcare profession courses. A number of those that are used in nurse education programmes for assessing theory and practice were identified in Box 5.3.

Action point 5.3 – How to assess standards of proficiency

From the list of assessment strategies identified in Box 5.3 and others that you have experience of, using the format below identify the different ways in which outcomes in each of the four domains of pre-registration programmes can be effectively assessed. You may wish to access all NMC standards of proficiency under the four domains to be more confident of your responses.

Domain	Most appropriate method of assessment	
	Theory	Practice
Professional and ethical practice		
Care management		
Personal and professional development		
Care delivery		

Practice teachers' competence includes the ability to design and implement a variety of assessment frameworks in the course of an assessment of standard of proficiency (NMC, 2008a). One way of doing this is by making decisions based on one or a range of methods of assessment that are valid, so as to make pass/fail decisions on students' competence with regard to each standard.

Practice teachers are of course expected to be fully cognisant of appropriate methods of assessment of the students' knowledge and comprehension as well, especially for students on specialist- or advanced-practice courses. However, unless the practice teacher is the course leader, they will generally only assess students' competence in clinical settings during practice placements. Box 5.5 suggests ways or frameworks for assessing students' competencies in each of the four domains of pre-registration nurse education (NMC, 2004b) and the domains of learning.

Box 5.5   NMC domains, how to assess theory and competence in the domains of learning

NMC domain	Domains of learning	Assessment method
Professional and ethical practice	Cognitive: theoretical knowledge	Seminar presentation Course portfolio

Care management	Cognitive and psychomotor	Essays Poster presentation Reflective account Portfolio Reflective account Work product
Personal and professional development	Cognitive and affective (attitude and interpersonal skills)	Checklist of interpersonal abilities Questioning Direct observation
Care delivery	Psychomotor	OSCE Direct observation and questioning Practice objectives Skill demonstration
	Practical knowledge	Work products Questioning

Various local terminologies and frameworks prevail in the identification of assessment strategies that are appropriate for specific competencies. For reflective accounts or a 'reflective wrapper', for instance, the student would be required to write an account that demonstrates a systematic reflection that is analytical and takes relevant knowledge (e.g. research) on the topic area into consideration. The reflection can be on an experience that has been problematic, enigmatic or an innovation, and needs to end with a summary of learning from the experience, and possibly an action plan.

Work products tend to refer to other forms of written work that the practice teacher might require the student to undertake such as a review of research on wound cleansing fluids, or in mental health the nature of emotions that can develop into aggressive outbursts. Furthermore, an assessment of competence should be undertaken through both direct observation in practice and evidence gained from indirect observation, as all assessment decisions must be evidence based, as discussed later in this chapter, as well as research on the assessment of professional knowledge and competence.

Furthermore, practice teachers can also utilise simulation for summative assessments where opportunities to demonstrate competence in practice are limited, for example a simulated case conference for child protection, case study presentations, or role plays. Additionally, new practice teachers might wish to seek advice and guidance from experienced practice teachers and other teachers when making complex judgements on encountering new situations, such as failing a student on their practice objectives.

Marking criteria

Students are informed of the specific pass/fail criteria for each assessment component very early on in their programmes. These criteria for individual assignments are determined locally by each university, and can also vary depending on the specific subject area of study, as noted earlier. Written essays tend to assess students' knowledge, comprehension, the application of concepts to practice, critical analysis, evaluation and synthesis. Reflective entries made by students in their portfolios tend to assess theoretical and practical knowledge, as well as the ability to reflect systematically. The likely items comprising the marking criteria for portfolios are identified in Box 5.6.

Box 5.6   Marking criteria and marker comment sheet for portfolios (post-graduate level)

Phoenix University

Post-graduate diploma in ....

COMMENTS ON PORTFOLIOS SUBMITTED FOR ASSESSMENT

Student's name:

Name of first marker: Recommendation: Pass/Fail

The portfolio has:

❖ A list of content showing the portfolio is well organised   Yes ☐   No ☐

❖ Evidence of achievement of all required/specified outcomes   Yes ☐   No ☐

❖ Evidence of practice skills   Yes ☐   No ☐

❖ Evidence of systematic reflection and learning from them   Yes ☐   No ☐

❖ Evidence of relevant reading, including research   Yes ☐   No ☐

❖ Evidence of critical analysis   Yes ☐   No ☐

❖ Evidence of coursework results   Yes ☐   No ☐

❖ A record of work experience attendance   Yes ☐   No ☐

❖ Meeting other professional bodies' specific requirements   Yes ☐   No ☐

First marker's comments: Date:

Second marker's/moderator's comments:

The items in the marking criteria sheet can be adapted and reproduced in the marker's comments or feedback sheet for a fuller impression of the quality of the work presented for assessment. The 'Yes' and 'No' columns in the comments sheet can be replaced by 'Achieved', 'Borderline' and 'Not Achieved'. In addition to the criteria on the comments sheet, markers may be issued with further guidelines for marking portfolios in order to address consistency across markers, and also for transparency and objectivity. These guidelines could include:

- Avoiding annotating the portfolio itself, and using a separate sheet for giving detailed feedback, by referring to specific pages of the portfolios.
- Grading the work, not the person.
- If referring to the person, using the second person 'you' form.
- Writing comments in a supportive and appreciative tone.
- Seeking assistance from others in the marking team or the course leader if you are uncertain about particular components of the portfolio.
- Indicating clearly what needs to be done in each component to improve the portfolio.
- Suggesting to the module/course leader which portfolios to moderate.

Universal marking criteria for portfolios can prove difficult to achieve as they are usually specific to course requirements and the year of study. Nonetheless, they should focus firmly on the theory–practice interface, and also demonstrate an appropriate level of critical analysis.

Spence and El-Ansari (2004) evaluated practice teachers' experiences of portfolio assessment of specialist community nursing practitioner students in which practice teachers reported that the source of portfolio evidence supplied by students included a record of discussions during supervision, other practitioners' reports and feedback from patients. They indicated that although the practice teacher's experience of portfolios was largely positive, the quality of portfolio evidence was varied.

However, Williams' (2003) research on the assessment of portfolios reveals that it is a sound and transparent approach to assessments, and that they were viewed as part of the learning process, and they encourage lifelong learning. Pitts et al. (1999), however, report that assessing portfolios is challenging and note that trained assessors can only achieve a certain degree of agreement (inter-rater reliability), even when judging portfolios against agreed criteria.

As with other theoretical components, portfolios can be double-marked blind, or second marked. First and second marking should be completed a few weeks before the Examinations and Assessment Board meeting to allow time for moderation. They are moderated by the course leader or another course-team member who is not involved in marking in order to achieve consistency across the team of markers. Comments and marks given by both markers can then be discussed at the moderating meeting when decisions can be made regarding any portfolio that needs further work to pass, and offering the student the chance ('rescue' feedback) to do this prior to the Examinations and Assessment Board meeting.

As with portfolios as an assessed component in healthcare education programmes, HEIs establish specific marking criteria for all other assessed components, such as those identified in Box 5.3, and how effective and 'fit for purpose' the set of criteria is can be ascertained through ongoing monitoring and research.

Service-user involvement in assessments

It could be argued that to ascertain how competently a healthcare profession student performs a clinical intervention, the assessor could consult the recipient of the intervention, that is the patient or service user. In fact, the NMC (2006b) and others indicate that where feasible patients or service users should be directly involved in the assessment of competence.

Rush and Barker (2006) and others explain ways of involving mental health service users in nurse education through enquiry-based learning, and in their research found that such an experience inspires students and contributes to the development of their understanding of mental health issues in both theory and practice.

However, as for an assessment of competence, in instances where patient or service users are involved, curriculum planners need to consider whether the assessment is:

- formative or summative
- for all clinical skills during the placement, or certain specified ones
- for the psychomotor domain, or the affective domain, i.e. attitude, interpersonal skills, as well.

Speers (2008) explored the views of a number of stakeholders (service users, lecturers, mentors, ex-students and student nurses) on the potential involvement of service users in the assessment of student mental-health nurses' competence in forming therapeutic relationships, and found that the service users interviewed had a largely positive attitude towards this potential development. Nurse participants were in favour in principle, but expressed reservations about how such a proposal could be implemented in practice. Speers recommends that patients' and service users' anonymity needs to be maintained, their consent obtained and the fairness of assessments ensured.

Assessing competence in pre-registration education

The practice teacher's role incorporates signing-off practice proficiency for finalist student nurses. To do so, the practice teacher assesses students on a set of 'essential skills' that have already been identified in the programme of study. Prior to reaching this stage a continuity of practice assessment is ensured through an assessment of clinical skills during each practice placement, and through an ongoing achievement record to confirm proficiency at a designated point in the programme. The essential skills identified for assessment are based on the NMC's (2004b) standards of proficiency for pre-registration nurse education.

Evidence of safe and effective practice is required at the appropriate academic levels, protected time for the assessment of essential skills is also required, and pass/fail decisions have to be reached.

Evidence-based assessment of safe and effective practice

As indicated variously, it is increasingly advocated that decisions on student competence should be evidence-based. Evidence-based assessment comprises evidence of the achievement of all the marking criteria issued by the HEI for an assessment of the knowledge component of the programme and the performance criteria for the assessment of competence. The total assessment strategy can include evidence of the student's performance from various sources such as patient-satisfaction reports, self-reports from students and observations and documentary reports from other colleagues and other professionals.

Students therefore need to be encouraged to keep a record of their learning experiences, identifying evidence to support the achievement of NMC outcomes and competencies and where further support and supervision are required. This record should be reviewed at intervals by their named practice teacher during their supervised practice experience to enable a discussion of strengths and areas for further learning. Students should therefore be given continual formative feedback on their performance so that the ultimate decision on their proficiency is not unexpected.

Consequently, practice teachers must also keep sufficient records of evidence to support and justify their decisions on whether a student is, or is not, competent. This can consist of an audit trail in support of their decisions.

Individual students present evidence of proficiency to their named practice teacher or sign-off mentor, based on the recorded evidence of an achievement of practice proficiency. Thus signing-off practice proficiency is a crucial role of practice teachers, as this is an NMC requirement, which the programme leader receives from sign-off mentors to present to the Examinations and Assessment Board for approval. If the student cannot provide evidence of proficiency by the end of the placement, then an extension or a repeat placement would be required to become proficient in the identified clinical skills.

Furthermore, the performance criteria (see Glossary) for the skill being assessed must be agreed beforehand, and therefore made transparent. The assessor makes pass/fail decisions for each skill for fitness for practice. In addition to the evidence presented by the student, the practice teacher should exercise their professional judgement when making pass/fail decisions, as advocated by Dowie and Elstein (1988).

The role of feedback in assessments

Following an assessment of the student's competence related to particular clinical skills, the practice teacher has to decide whether to award a pass or a fail to the student for the skill assessed. However, before announcing the result, the practice teacher has to provide comments to the student on the competence level displayed. One of the most significant reasons for providing comments is to present guidance on how to improve and enhance their performance of the particular clinical interventions, or transfer the skill to other clinical situations. This is because all assessments should incorporate an element of learning as an integral feature, as also advocated by Quinn and Hughes (2007), for instance.

One of the roles of feedback is to fill the gap between the expected level of performance, and the actual performance displayed. Feedback to students can also constitute redress for a situation where the student is harbouring misconceptions based on comparing their performance with those of more senior healthcare professionals, or with a weaker performance that they might have witnessed. It should provide the student with practical advice that can increase their motivation to learn, and is also a significant feature of an effective learning ethos.

Feedback should be given continuously (i.e. formative feedback) throughout the learning experience (e.g. the practice placement), which is different from summative feedback, which in turn is given at specific points during the place-ment when pass or fail decisions are made and documented. Rogers (2007) suggests that we learn from our successes, not just our failings, which is done by ascertaining which of our actions were the ingredients for success, that is those performed correctly. There should therefore be more emphasis on the positive components of the performance, and they should be given promptly after the performance.

Various guidelines on how to give useful feedback can be found in the education literature. The 'sandwich method' is widely advocated whereby after asking the student how well they feel they performed the clinical skill, the learning facilitator initially states the areas of strength in the student's performance, which are followed by aspects that can be improved and further developed, and ended by highlighting further strengths. Box 5.7 identifies good practice guidelines for giving effective feedback.

Box 5.7   Good practice guidelines for giving effective feedback

ACTIONS	RATIONALES
Give feedback promptly after the performance, and calmly	To alleviate student uncertainty and suspense
Ensure ample time and privacy for giving feedback	So that the feedback can be given in full, not partially
Ask the student how well they feel they performed the skill	To drive their attention away from any anxiety they might be experiencing, which comprises self-assessment, and focuses attention on the 'performance criteria'
Praise the student on the actions that they have undertaken correctly and efficiently, using factual details	Positive points reinforce correct practices, but starting with weaknesses can lead the student to believe they have failed and are unable to take any further informationin accurately
Point out the actions that they show weaknesses in	This can also direct the learner to areas of further learning
Indicate whether they are being awarded a pass or a fail, or a specific grade, and why	So that the student understands the reasoning underpinning the decision, and can progress on to further learning

Do not extrapolate the weaknesses in their performance as components of their personality	To avoid suggesting that the weaknesses shown are personality traits that cannot be changed
Ensure feedback is constructive, i.e. when indicating weaknesses, suggest alternative ways in which the weaknesses can be rectified	Because the assessment is also a medium for identifying further learning
Feel free to take a little time out to reflect or consult a team member if unsure of any aspect of the assessment	This prevents a rushed decision, especially in borderline situations, and can prevent making an incorrect decision
Be sensitive to, and act on, the emotions being felt by the student during the feedback session	Because not all weaknesses need to be elaborated on in detail if the student is becoming distraught
Provide the recipient with opportunities to ask for clarifications	To ensure the effectiveness of the feedback and to reinforce the main messages
You must feel responsible for the feedback you give	Because this will guide the student's subsequent learning
Complete documentations as discussed, and sign and date as expected	To ensure the actions taken are recorded
The final stages of the feedback must take a strong positive tone	To ensure the student is encouraged and motivated to continue learning

Additionally, the concept 'feed-forward' has been advocated, which constitutes a strategy for enabling students to make more effective use of assessment feedback. Feed-forward comprises planned discussions wherein students actively engage with the assessment criteria and understand them to be able to produce improved subsequent work. However, for this to happen, firstly, feed-forward must be embedded in the course curriculum; and, second, when marking assignments, the focus of the feedback should involve moving away from merely grading and justifying the grade to enable learning from the feedback comments.

Established local protocols guides the practice teacher as to which course team member (e.g. link tutor or personal tutor) to inform if the student displays unsafe practice. Unsafe and ineffective patient or service-user care constitutes unethical practice, which is discussed in Chapter 6.

Assessing specialist and advanced practice

As indicated at the beginning of this chapter, probably the most critical component of the practice teacher role is the assessment of students' specialist or advanced practice proficiency in order to ascertain safe and effective practice, for example for

SCPHNs. This can include cross-professional assessment, that is an assessment of the competence of other health profession students. Assessments have to determine fitness for practice as well as fitness for purpose and an award at specialist and advanced practice levels.

Specialist or advanced knowledge and competence in your field of practice

The standards of proficiency for particular specialist and advanced practice areas are usually identified by the profession's regulatory body. These standards inform the set of practice competencies that students on specialist or advanced practice programmes have to achieve and demonstrate a capability to perform.

Action point 5.4 – Assessing specialist and advanced practice

Consider the outcomes or standards that students on specialist or advanced practice programmes in your specialist area should achieve to qualify as specialist or advanced practitioners. Subsequently, as with the exercise suggested for assessing pre-registration programme standards of proficiency in Action Point 5.1, consider and make notes on the assessment strategies that can be used to assess safe and effective practice for these outcomes.

Canham (2001) explored how practice educators classify specialist-practitioner student practice, and found that many students overestimate or underestimate their practice achievements, as perceived by the practice educators. There were also concerns about the timing of assessments and the applied terminology, and Canham concluded that the role of the HEI should include ensuring essential preparation and ongoing support for practice educators in a tri-partite assessment process.

Assessing safe and effective specialist or advanced practice skills

Students on specialist or advanced practice programmes are assessed on their specialist and advanced practice knowledge and competence using a booklet of practice competencies or practice outcomes. These competencies are usually derived from national standards such as the NMC's (2005a) domains, or the Royal College of Nursing's (2008) *RCN Competencies: Advanced Nurse Practitioners - an RCN Guide to the Advanced Nurse Practitioner Role, Competencies and Programme Accreditation,* and on research (e.g. Gardner et al., 2007). The RCN's guide details ANP competencies that are akin to the NMC's under the domains identified in Box 1.4 in Chapter 1.

The number of competencies varies according to the amount of professional activity involved, and the first domain 'Assessment and management of patient health/illness status', for instance, consists of 32 competencies, while 'The nurse–patient relationship' has ten.

For the assessment of students on SCPHN programmes, the NMC (2004a) details the outcomes *Standards of Proficiency for Specialist Community Public Health Nurses* – see Table 3.1 in Chapter 3. A case study illustrates the assessment strategy that was implemented to ascertain the achievement of NMC outcomes for practice teachers.

Case study

HA is a well-qualified and an experienced mental health nurse who gained a BA (Hons) in Psychology and Sociology and thereafter the mental health nursing NMC registerable qualification. She has attended a range of post-qualifying short courses as part of her professional development since, and took the practice teacher course as part of the MSc in the Advancing Practice programme. HA is currently a deputy ward manager in acute mental-health services and has substantial experience of mentoring healthcare and social-care students. HA did not have a specialist mental health practice student on placement in her department during the six months duration of the practice teacher course, nor a qualified practice teacher in her workplace to facilitate her development as a practice teacher and to assess her on the NMC's domains and outcomes for practice teachers.

To enable HA to achieve these course requirements, HA was supported by the mental health PEF (with NMC approved teacher qualification), who had one-to-one supervision discussions with HA in the practice setting, utilising questioning as one of the methods of assessment, with the onus being on HA to supply evidence of the achievement of the NMC outcomes, which included two reflective accounts. HA was observed facilitating learning for mental health nurses on short learning beyond initial registration courses. Her skills in assessing student competence and her leadership related to specialist practice were achieved under the supervision of mental health lecturers in the university setting with students on a cognitive behaviour therapy course, through the utilisation of role plays, simulation-based assessment exercises and questioning.

Cross-professional assessment

With the advent and widespread implementation of inter-professional working and learning also arrived the legitimation of cross-professional assessment (e.g. NMC, 2008a). This involves an assessment of student competence by an appropriate member of another healthcare profession, or a social-care profession, usually when the student is on a practice placement with them. However, the named practice teacher must verify and countersign the practice competency based on discussions with the subsidiary assessor.

Examples include pharmacists assessing nurses on nurse prescribing courses, doctors assessing endoscopy specialist nurses, and so on. Similarly, nurses and midwives are involved in assessing students on other healthcare and social care-profession courses, for example medical students.

Furthermore, the practice teacher has to comply with due regard, i.e. to be the named practice teacher for students on the same branch and specialism as the student (NMC, 2008a).

Maintaining academic and professional standards

Validity and reliability of assessments

An assessment of both professional knowledge and competence needs to measure what it set out to measure in the first place, which makes it a 'valid' assessment. If when the assessment is conducted again by either the same or another assessor and the same result is awarded for the same quality of performance, then the assessment meets the reliability criteria as well. Intra- and inter-assessor reliability is discussed in Chapter 8.

Maintaining national standards

To ensure standards are maintained in the assessment of students' knowledge and competence, assessments are conducted by designated course team members, which are then moderated, and subsequently scrutinised by external examiners. Final pass/fail decisions are corroborated at the Examinations and Assessment Board's meeting.

In the UK, the academic standards of professional courses are established and monitored in various ways. For nursing courses for instance, a number of organisations currently have to, or might want to, appraise whether the proposed and already established university professional courses meet their standards and requirements. These organisations include:

- The Nursing and Midwifery Council.
- The local Strategic Health Authority.
- The Quality Assurance Agency for Higher Education.
- The Health Professions Council.
- The university's own quality monitoring department.
- Skills for Health.
- The external peer-reviewer mechanism, e.g. by external examiners.

The QAA's qualification descriptors, which can be utilised to ascertain academic standard at the third year of a degree-level programme, were presented in Box 5.1. The ultimate criteria for passing students are that they can demonstrate fitness for practice and purpose and award for specialist and advanced practice.

Other organisations that might be involved include the Higher Education Academy for a post-graduate certificate in education or equivalent courses, medicine and pharmacy organisations for non-medical prescribing courses, and so on.

Research on the assessment of competencies

Research on the assessment of professional knowledge and competence is regularly published in journal articles and in monographs and reports, and presented at relevant national and international conferences. For instance, Tee and Jowett (2009) explored the extent to which healthcare profession programmes achieved 'fitness for practice' at the School of Nursing at one UK university, and concluded that such explorations with a focus on minimum risks to patients and service-users raise students' awareness of their professional responsibilities and integrity.

Research on assessment methods such as OSCEs, for example, includes a study by Major (2005) who explored progress on the role of OSCEs in pre-registration curricula and concluded that it is not a bandwagon, but a form of assessment that has evolved over time into a valid and reliable way of assessing student competence. OSCEs were initially used in medical courses, and are now used in several healthcare profession courses, for example in rehabilitation courses and those in physiotherapy. OSCEs are crucial to the learning process as they encourage healthcare profession students to adopt a critical and holistic view of their practice and enable the acquisition of essential skills.

Byrne and Smyth (2008) conducted a qualitative study of lecturers' experiences and perspectives of using OSCEs, and concluded that nurse educators should recognise both the potential and the contribution of OSCEs to the curriculum and increase students' exposure to this assessment strategy.

For learning beyond initial registration, Khattab and Rawlings (2008), for instance, explored the assessment of nurse-practitioner students' clinical competence using a modified OSCE assessment method that was developed to standardise the evaluation of examining skills by using healthy student volunteers to simulate patients. They indicate that the modified OSCE is also being used successfully as a tool for formative and summative assessment, as a learning resource, and as a basis for physical examination assessments to identify gaps and weaknesses in clinical skills.

Brookes (2007) reports on an assessment of competence by OSCEs for students on nurse prescribing courses. The implementation of this method of assessment also resulted in recommendations such as piloting the OSCE scenarios before presenting them to students as summative assessments, joint assessment by two assessors, and ensuring that transparent pass/fail criteria are established beforehand.

Another study on assessments that was based on a recognition that students have different strengths, weaknesses, learning styles and preferred modes of assessment entailed a project that afforded students on pre-registration, and on CPD modules, a choice of modes of assessment (Garside et al., 2009). The project was systematically designed and managed giving pre-registration students a choice between an essay, a presentation and a seen written examination, and CPD students a choice between designing a teaching package, posters, and so on. Garside et al. report that such choices were well received by students whilst also meeting quality assurance requirements.

Conclusion

The focus of Chapter 5 has been on the assessment of the knowledge and competence of healthcare professionals as students on specialist and advanced practice programmes. Essential assessment frameworks were examined in order to ensure safe and effective practice, how pass/fail decisions are reached, signing-off practice proficiency and cross-professional assessment. It therefore covered:

- The contemporary nature of assessments, what assessments are, the general aims and principles of assessments, in the context of the practice teacher role, an exploration of the various reasons for assessing students, and how to assess specialist and advanced knowledge and competencies, implementing a variety of assessment frameworks, taxonomy levels for assessing practice and theory, and research on the assessment of competence.
- Assessing competence in pre-registration education, which includes an evidence-based assessment of safe and effective practice, signing-off practice proficiency, the role of professional judgement and giving effective feedback.
- Assessing specialist and advanced practice knowledge and competence in your field of practice, assessing students on SCPHN, SPQ and ANP programmes using different methods of assessment for safe and effective practice, and cross-professional assessment.
- Maintaining academic and professional standards in assessment and accountability, which incorporate national guidelines and standards, and the validity and reliability of assessments.

Nursing and other healthcare professions are practice-based vocations that require learning clinical intervention skills, and their students' competence in each skill needs to be assessed and documented by appropriately qualified and up-to-date healthcare professionals. Chapter 6 will address the practice teacher's responsibilities and accountability in their roles as specialist or advanced practitioners, and in the supervision of learning and assessment.

6

The Practice Teacher's Accountability

Introduction

The preceding chapters of this book have explored several areas of practice teaching, namely the reasons for, and the scope of, practice teaching and learning, establishing and managing professional working relationships, facilitating learning and the assessment of generic, specialist and advanced clinical practice knowledge and competence, and the practice teacher as an evidence-based practitioner and practice developer.

In Chapter 6, the focus is on the practice teacher's responsibilities and accountability in specialist and advanced practice, and in the supervision of learning and the assessment of students on pre- and post-qualifying healthcare courses. Assessment and accountability encompass the decision to pass or fail students on practice competencies, considering the justification and ethical implications of these decisions, and also ways of managing students who are underachieving.

Chapter outcomes

On completion of this chapter you should be able to:

1 Identify the reasons for examining the practice teacher's accountability, and demonstrate knowledge and understanding of accountability and inherent concepts, such as types of accountability, as well as the role of professional regulatory bodies.
2 Evaluate the responsibilities and accountability of practice teaching, including components that the practice teacher is accountable for, such as safe and effective specialist and advanced practice, for teaching and assessing specialist and advanced practice students, and for signing off practice proficiency.
3 Critically evaluate the frameworks, principles and processes of assessment of practice at pre- and post-registration levels, with accountability, confirming that students have or have not achieved their practice competencies, and managing failing students.
4 Enunciate the critical significance of ethical practice in practice teaching, and ethical competence in assessing clinical skills, including when signing off standards of proficiency.

Why explore the practice teacher's accountability?

There are several reasons for exploring the practice teacher's accountability. What the term accountability means is examined first in this chapter, then followed by an appraisal of specific components of work roles that healthcare professionals are accountable for, and to whom, and also the professional regulation of healthcare professions.

In addition to the above perspectives on accountability, the NMC (2008a: 53) also indicates (under the domain 'Assessment and accountability') that the practice teacher's accountability includes managing 'failing students so that they may enhance their performance and capabilities for safe and effective practice or be able to understand their failure and the implications of this for their future'. Clearly the practice teacher's responsibility in ascertaining their students' capability for safe and effective practice has very important implications, as if they award a pass to students who are not competent, then this is also unethical practice on their part and, much more importantly, their student could engage in unethical clinical practice through faulty care delivery, as also noted by Gopee (2008b).

It is also unethical in that this action can inadvertently mislead the student and future healthcare professional into believing that they are competent when they are not. However, from another angle, the NMC indicates that the practice teacher must help the student to understand the implications of their failure for their future. This statement can imply that the student should be helped to realise that if they have tried their best but are still unable to develop competence in required clinical skills, then they may need to identify more achievable and realistic objectives and constitute an action plan, and even reconsider their position with regard to nursing as their career path.

Additionally, Duffy's (2004) 'failing to fail' report recommends that programmes preparing healthcare professionals for supporting learning and assessment should address the issue of accountability and the potential consequences of passing students without adequate evidence of competence. This is so as to protect the public from unsafe and ineffective practice that can result in harm to patients. Protecting the public is the primary role of the NMC through the investigation of reported incompetent practice.

The practice teacher is usually also a mentor on the live mentor database held by the relevant local healthcare trust, and would already be competent in the NMC (2008a) practice teacher outcomes. However, these outcomes refer in particular to supervising and facilitating learning for students on specialist and advanced practice courses, and therefore to the acquisition of specialist skills in areas such as emergency care and neonatal nursing, or for health screening for a specific at-risk group of individuals, undertaking endoscopic procedures, or managing a critically ill baby who is on a ventilator, as appropriate.

Some of the principles (linked to theories) of managing a specific group of individuals are published in the form of standards listed in National Service Frameworks (NSF) (such as *National Service Framework for Older People* (DH, 2001b)) that documents key standards for this age group, and clinical guidelines published by relevant organisations such as NICE. Integration of these principles or theories with practice entails implementing the standards in the appropriate

NSF or clinical guideline into day-to-day care delivery, and doing so with the resources that are available. It then incorporates reflective practice.

What is accountability?

Like all nurses, practice teachers normally encounter the term accountability primarily in the purview of the NMC's (2008d) code of professional practice, which begins by stating that 'As a professional, you are personally accountable for actions and omissions in your practice and must always be able to justify your decisions' (p. 1).

Action point 6.1 – Defining accountability

Based on your professional experience in healthcare over a number of years as a healthcare professional, compile your own definition of accountability as you understand it.

Accountability for professional practice refers to the practitioner being able to provide reasonable rationales for their actions (and omissions). Following an analysis of the evolution of the term accountability, Jacobs (2004) indicates that the term does not exist in many languages, including European ones, having instead terms like answerability and reporting. Jacobs indicates that the term has become multi-faceted and that makes a simple definition of the term 'meaningless'.

Dictionaries indicate that being accountable refers to being 'liable to be called to account or to answer for responsibilities, discharge of duties, and conduct'. As healthcare professionals we are both accountable and responsible for our clinical activities. The two concepts can be distinguished from each other in a number of ways. We are responsible for all our activities and behaviours, mostly those that we personally choose to do or adopt, but we are accountable for those that we are allocated or assigned to do during the course of our duties, and in healthcare for every activity that we engage in that can affect others.

Students, for instance, have a responsibility to ensure they perform clinical interventions in accordance with the healthcare organisation's policies, procedures and clinical guidelines, but it is their clinically based teacher who is accountable for ensuring that the student performs the intervention accordingly, safely and effectively, and in accordance with the NMC's (2008d) code of practice. The practice teacher therefore may delegate the responsibility for caring for particular patients or service users or for particular clinical interventions, but they are accountable for ensuring that the student performs the delegated responsibilities to the required standard.

Consequently, we can have various responsibilities but accountability for only certain specific ones. According to the dictionary, to be responsible refers to 'being capable of fulfilling an obligation or trust; reliable, trustworthy'. A definition of accountability in the context of nursing accountability is that it is a 'preparedness to explain and justify one's intentions, acts and omissions in the context of team-working and organisational demands and constraints' (University of Surrey, 2008: 2).

Lewis and Batey (1982) are widely cited for identifying accountability as meaning the fulfilment of a formal obligation to disclose to referent others the purposes, principles, procedures, relationships, results or expenditures for which one has authority. However, in a study conducted on behalf of the RCN, Savage and Moore (2004) indicate that attempting to define accountability by combining and sequencing inherent concepts to explain the concept is a futile exercise as it comprises diverse meanings to different individuals. They suggest that accountability can mean both to be 'counted on' (in the sense of being dependable) and 'being able to be counted' (to report poor practice). Pursuing her analysis of accountability in nursing, Jacobs (2004) further argues that accountability is an elusive and complex concept that is, on the other hand, closely linked to professionalism.

Watson (2004: 38) also firmly links accountability with professionalism, indicating that it is 'the hallmark of a profession', and Jacobs (2004) notes that professional identity is constructed at two levels, which are: (i) externally, i.e. in terms of the professional status awarded by society; and (ii) internally, i.e. in terms of the individual's own perception of their self as a professional in their chosen vocation.

Furthermore, the broadness of the topic can be illustrated by considering, for instance, the variety of aspects of accountability on the General Medical Council's (2008) website, such as the scope and extent of accountability, and accountability:

- for practitioners' conduct through their management
- for withholding or withdrawing care
- in life-prolonging treatments
- in multi-disciplinary and multi-agency teams
- for lines of management
- for managers' accountability
- to the GMC for clinical interventions
- for good medical practice – when delegating, when managing finances, when referring.

Who are practice teachers accountable to, and what for?

There are various authorities and personnel to whom all nurses are accountable for their work, and even their non-work activities.

Action point 6.2 – Accountable to whom?

Consider your accountability for both care delivery and practice teacher roles, and make notes on all the personnel and authorities to whom you are accountable for your patient-related actions and decisions.

Deducing from various perspectives, two key facets of accountability emerge, that is accountable to whom and the modes of accountability. As for the first facet, it is quite well documented that we are accountable to (and for) the patient, under both civil and criminal laws, to our profession, to the general public and to our professional regulatory body, as well as to our employer. In brief detail the areas of accountability that we could be asked to defend or explain are:

- the patient – 'duty of care', and able to justify actions and decisions (under civil law)
- ourselves as individuals – for our own standards
- our employer – through our contract of employment (under employment law)
- the professional regulatory body – for professional standards
- our colleagues – e.g. medical, nurse peers
- to our profession – as seen, for example, by Royal College of Nursing (Savage and Moore, 2004)
- society – for promoting health
- the public and the patient's family – under criminal law.

The reason for suggesting that defining accountability is problematic is also because of the various dimensions and modes of accountability. Savage and Moore identify diverse areas of accountability such as fiscal, process, programme, priorities, social, ethical, legal and professional accountability. Our various modes of accountability as healthcare professionals are as follows:

- personal accountability: related to personal values, philosophies and standards, commitment to care
- professional accountability: for actions during the course of one's duty – to colleagues, employer, professional regulatory body
- managerial accountability: for management decisions, e.g. appropriate delegation of tasks, duties, and authority
- budgetary accountability: when budgets are allocated to the clinician/nurse manager – for an efficient use of resources
- political accountability: being answerable for actions that impact on society
- clinical governance accountability: for continuous improvement of quality of care and treatment, clinical audits and best practice guidelines.

The dimensions of accountability can be illustrated hierarchically as preconditions of accountability – see Figure 6.1. which indicates that to be in a position to be accountable, the healthcare professional must be competent to practice, that is have the necessary knowledge, skills and values, and the external resources (material, equipment, etc.) in the first place. They must also be afforded an appropriate degree of responsibility, authority and autonomy.

Professional accountability and professional regulation

Healthcare professionals are of course accountable for their clinical practice. Instances of incompetent practice result in the healthcare professional being called to appear before the NMC's misconduct committee, whenceforth they can be exonerated, suspended, cautioned or struck off the NMC's professional register. Reports on

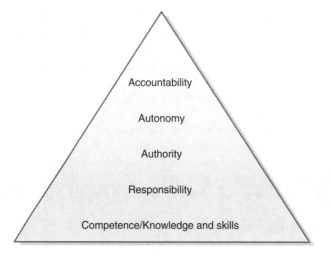

Figure 6.1   *Dimensions of accountability*

instances (or case studies) of misconduct hearings are regularly published on the professional regulatory bodies' websites, such as those of the NMC and HPC which identify individuals who end up in these categories. Often the reason for this is a breach of a certain clause of the NMC's (2008d) code of practice, which is periodically reviewed and adjusted, based on a process that includes consultation with nurses, midwives and the public, and when a new edition is published, a copy is sent to each nurse and midwife on the NMC register.

The NMC is the professional regulator for nurses and midwives. Professional regulation for other healthcare and social care professions is currently undertaken by the HPC and the GSSC respectively. The HPC (2006) details ten healthcare profession regulators in the UK and four 'Social Care' regulators (constituting one for each UK country), which can be viewed on the HPC website.

Various areas of further work are underway to implement this provision, which also involves a revalidation for doctors through portfolio evidence. Because of these and other issues, the government is reviewing the regulation of medical and all related health professions, which is embodied in its White Paper, *Trust, Assurance and Safety – The Regulation of Health Professionals in the 21st Century* (DH, 2007a). The Council for Healthcare Regulatory Excellence (CHRE), which is an independent body accountable to parliament, already scrutinises and oversees the work of health-professions' regulators. However, Savage and Moore (2004) also note that there is ambiguity in the literature and the clinical area about the nature and extent of the accountability of different professional groups. They note that many of the professional conduct cases appearing before the NMC, for instance, arise from nurses' uncertainty or lack of awareness about their accountability.

Additionally, the professional regulation refers to the focused activities of an organisation that is set up with the specific remit to develop, enforce and monitor standards of practice for the particular profession(s) it regulates. These standards include individual nurses and midwives being required to provide evidence of professional updating (post-registration education and practice – PREP) as a condition for being permitted to continue practising as a nurse, that is revalidation. This has proved somewhat problematic, as identified by Gopee (2001).

The CHRE comprises a mechanism that was established by parliament in 2003 to ensure consistency and good practice in healthcare regulation. It is an independent statutory body that oversees the performance of the nine healthcare regulators in the United Kingdom, including the NMC, HPC and GMC. It forms part of a more robust and overarching mechanism that is being developed through the government's White Paper *Trust, Assurance and Safety – The Regulation of Health Professionals in the 21st Century* (DH, 2007a), which itself comprises a major development that outlines how healthcare professions are to be regulated in the future. It takes into account the recommendations of major reviews of professional regulation, such as one by the Chief Medical Officer entitled *Good Doctors, Safer Patients* (DH, 2006c), and another entitled *The Regulation of the Non-Medical Healthcare Professions* (DH, 2007e). Progress in the work of the CHRE and developments related to the White Paper are regularly published on relevant sections of the Department of Health website.

Because certain weaknesses related to professional regulation have surfaced over recent years, the aim of the abovementioned White Paper is to address these weaknesses by implementing a more effective regulatory mechanism. The DH (2008g) indicates that the five principles for good regulation are that they are:

- transparent
- accountable
- proportionate
- consistent, and
- targeted where action is needed.

The DH also identifies and provides details of 12 key principles for the development of non-medical revalidation – see Box 6.1 for the areas addressed by these principles. Detailed explanation of these principles is given in the DH (2008g) document. Moreover, the NMC (2008a) indicates that it is also awaiting developments in the implementation of this White Paper to ascertain ways of registering ANP qualifications on the NMC register. The NMC has already published its mapping of the NMC approved competencies for advanced practice against the *NHS KSF* dimensions (NMC, 2006a), but implementation is pending until the Department of Health's decision on the regulation of healthcare professions, and the Privy Council's response to the NMC's request to record ANP qualifications on a sub-part of the nurses' part of the NMC's professional register.

Box 6.1   Key principles for the development of non-medical revalidation

- Consistency
- Professional standards
- Remediation
- Equality
- Integration
- UK-wide

(Continued)

(Continued)

- Patient and public involvement
- Continuing professional development
- Quality assurance
- Demonstrating benefits
- Information
- Incremental introduction

Almost all nurses always comply with statutory legislation and legal requirements, and the vast majority act in accordance with the professional code of practice, and consistently meet the professional standards expected by the public. Approximately 0.2 per cent of registered nurses and midwives, though, have their conduct investigated by the NMC through 'Fitness to Practice' hearings. Of the cases that are referred to the NMC (2008e) there are different outcomes for different incidents, and under *Sanctions and Disposal Options*, the NMC details the likely outcomes of misconduct hearings – see Table 6.1.

Table 6.1   *NMC's outcomes of cases of misconduct hearings*

	Investigating Committee Panel (IC)	Conduct and Competence Committee (CCC)	Health Committee Panel (HC)
Striking off Order		✓	✓
Removal – incorrect or fraudulent entry	✓		
Caution Order (1 to 5 years)		✓	✓
Conditions of Practice Order (up to 3 years)		✓	✓
Interim Suspension Order (up to 18 months)	✓	✓	✓
Interim Conditions of Practice Order (up to 18 months)	✓	✓	✓
Suspension Order (up to 12 months)		✓	✓

Source: NMC, 2008f

Various professional regulatory bodies regulate their own healthcare professions, but when on occasion alleged weaknesses in their mechanisms surface, some of these are made public. The NMC's revalidation mechanism has been criticised for not addressing CPD adequately, and for the audit of professional profiles as being inconsistent, and therefore these audits were subsequently suspended in 2008 till further notice.

Furthermore, in 2008, a Member of Parliament accused the NMC of being racist and using bullying tactics in its operations, which led to an investigation by the CHRE, who found the allegation to have substance. It also found poor leadership as well as other weaknesses such as extensive delays in misconduct hearings. This led to the resignation of the NMC's then Chief Executive and President who were deemed accountable for these weaknesses, and to the CHRE requesting specific changes to be made.

A later report by the CHRE (2008b) indicated that the NMC manages 'fitness to practise' (cases of misconduct) less effectively than other health profession regulators, in that it takes much longer to conclude a case from the time the allegation is received than the other regulators do. However, the NMC was commended for its work on standards and guidance and its registration processes, and the progress that the NMC has made in improving its performance over time was acknowledged.

It is increasingly well recognised that robust professional regulation is a crucial component of healthcare professionals' work activities. During this decade professional regulation guidelines and requirements have increasingly been tightened. The DH (2008e), for instance, states that doctors are required to renew their professional registration every five years. Those for non-medical professions are also about to be established.

Issues related to accountability and responsibilities surface every so often, and if they remain disputed, they are eventually resolved in a court of law. For example, *Nursing Standard News* (2008b: 8) reported on instance when a High Court judge overturned a ruling by the NMC who had found an accident and emergency nurse guilty of misconduct when a patient died in her department, but the judge ruled that although the individual had been the most senior nurse on the ward that night, she had not been personally responsible for the patient's care. The judge called for nurses to be given clear guidance on their responsibility for their colleagues' work.

Kitson (1993) and the NMC (2008e) recommend moving beyond professional accountability towards personal accountability, which can be achieved internally and externally – internally by peer review, professional supervision and personal accountability; and externally by peer-review, policies and authoritative guidelines, hierarchical accountability, and so on.

However, with the advent of clinical governance in 1997 in UK healthcare, it is both the individual healthcare professional who is accountable, and also the healthcare organisation. Clinical governance refers to continuous and co-ordinated quality monitoring and improvement. It is, however, also useful to note that corporate governance, as the predecessor of clinical governance in UK healthcare, was also based on the principles that organisations having to be accountable have an absolute standard of honesty (probity), and their activities have to be sufficiently transparent to be able to warrant trust (Tilley and Watson, 2004: 68). Clinical governance therefore makes organisations and individuals jointly accountable for clinical activities, which therefore require appropriate structures and local culture (such as no-blame culture) for this to happen.

Responsibilities and accountability of a practice teacher

A practice teacher is therefore accountable for safe and effective specialist and advanced practice, for teaching and assessing specialist or advanced practice students, as well as for signing off practice proficiency. They also have a responsibility for keeping up to date with their practice and ensuring it is evidence-based.

What is the practice teacher accountable for?

Besides the multiple dimensions of nurses' accountability discussed in the preceding sections, there are specific components that practice teachers are accountable for. The NMC (2008a: 22) indicates that practice teachers are responsible and accountable for all components of their roles, including:

- organising and co-ordinating learning activities, primarily in practice learning environments for pre-registration students, and those intending to register as a SCPHN and specialist practice qualifications where this is a local requirement
- assessing total performance – including skills, attitudes and behaviours.

The eight domains (NMC, 2008a) in which the practice teacher has to be competent encompass the hands-on care component, the management component and the teaching component of the practice teacher's work activities, and also implicitly comprise their areas of accountability. In particular, the practice teacher is accountable for their own competence in all 26 NMC (2008a) outcomes for practice teachers under the eight domains, from the steps they take to establish an effective relationship with students, to providing leadership in planning learning experiences for students and prioritising work to accommodate them, as well as being a competent, safe and effective clinician. The various components of healthcare professionals' work function, along with details of inherent activities, are also identified in the *NHS KSF* (DH, 2004a: 6) core and specific dimensions of NHS posts (as detailed in Chapter 1), which also comprise areas of accountability for practice teachers.

Consequently, practice teachers are accountable for safe and effective specialist or advanced practice, as well as for teaching and assessing specialist or advanced practice students. As a specialist or advanced practice clinician, the practice teacher is accountable for a greater range of clinical interventions than registrants who are not. They engage in more expanded roles. Hichen (2008) notes, for instance, that at one UK healthcare trust the accountability of modern matrons is accentuated in that they have to report on a weekly review on 18 criteria that include MRSA and clostridium difficile rates, and pressure ulcer levels.

Accountability for signing off practice proficiency

As briefly noted in Chapter 5, the practice teacher's role includes signing-off proficiency for pre-registration nurses during their final practice placement and for students on post-qualifying specialist or advanced practice courses. For pre-registration students, the NMC (2008a: Foreword) indicates that the practice teacher as a sign-off mentor '. . . must make the final assessment of practice and confirm that the required proficiencies for entry to the register have been achieved'. For students on specialist and advanced practice programmes leading to a recordable qualification on the NMC register, the sign-off practice teacher performs the final assessment of practice and confirms that the student has achieved the required proficiencies.

For the practice teacher to achieve sign-off status they need additional educational preparation, after which their new status is annotated accordingly in the local register of mentors and practice teachers. For the practice teacher to fulfil this role, the sign-off practice teacher must fulfil further criteria (NMC, 2008a) which are identified in Box 6.2.

Box 6.2   Criteria for a sign-off mentor

- Identified on the local register as a sign-off mentor or a practice teacher.
- Registered on the same part of the register.
- Working in the same field of practice as that in which the student intends to qualify.
- Has clinical currency and capability in the field in which the student is being assessed.
- Has a working knowledge of current programme requirements, practice assessment strategies and relevant changes in education and practice for the student they are assessing.
- Has an understanding of the NMC registration requirements and the contribution they make to the achievement of these requirements.
- Has an in-depth understanding of their accountability to the NMC for the decision they must make to pass or fail a student when assessing proficiency requirements at the end of a programme.
- Has been supervised on at least three occasions for signing off proficiency by an existing sign-off mentor

The practice teacher is responsible and accountable for making the final sign-off of proficiency in practice at the end of the three-year nurse education programme, confirming that the student has successfully completed all the practice requirements. The practice teacher should therefore be able to justify their decisions in signing-off the achievement of proficiency, as signing-off proficiency includes an accountability for reviewing students' documentation and ensuring that on the basis of the evidence provided they have met all the standards of proficiency. A working knowledge of a student's programme and assessment requirements, and an in-depth understanding of their own professional accountability when assessing proficiency, are therefore essential.

Sign-off proficiency results and documentation are eventually presented at the HEI's Examinations and Assessment Board, and when a student has met all the course requirements, including the criteria for 'good health and good character', then they can apply to have their name recorded on the NMC's register.

Signing-off proficiency comprises a declaration that the assessee meets the 'fitness for practice' criteria, and the practice teacher therefore must not sign any proficiency as a pass if insufficient evidence of competence is presented by the student. The consequences of 'failing to fail' are highlighted by Duffy (2004) and Gopee (2008b), for instance.

Practice teachers are accountable for all clinical interventions that they perform in the course of caring for patients or service users. They are also responsible for their own CPD in all domains of the role, and therefore need to ensure they are up to date with the criteria identified in Box 1.1 in Chapter 1. These are discussed further in Chapter 8.

Accountability and under-achieving students

When assessing competence in standards of proficiency for pre-registration student nurses and for post-qualifying students on specialist or advanced practice educational programmes, the practice teacher's aim is to ascertain fitness for practice, making pass/fail decisions, and managing under-achieving students.

Managing under-achieving students

Generally, practice placements are allocated to students well in advance, and a fairly detailed timetable is planned prior to the start of the placement. Practice objectives are identified very early in the placement, and both student and practice teacher monitor progress with the achievement of these objectives informally and continually. At times, students will experience difficulty achieving competencies by the pre-set dates, and the practice teacher needs to be aware of these difficulties, and thereafter follow the agreed protocol of actions.

The RCN (2007c), for instance, indicates that if a student is not achieving the necessary competencies as expected, then the mentor should take the following actions:

- meet with the student as soon as possible to discuss this issue, and ensure the student knows the reason for the meeting
- inform the HEI contact person, associate mentor and clinical placement/practice facilitator so that both you (the mentor) and the student have independent support available
- clarify the area of weakness and advise how to progress
- form a realistic action plan to address the issues, and set deadlines
- work closely with the student
- arrange for the student to work with other assessors to ensure fairness
- make provision for any extra support or opportunities to improve within the practice area that the student may require
- keep careful notes of all discussions and incidents.

Detailed protocols are established locally by universities, which tend to incorporate national guidelines such those by the RCN, and specific ones such as when the practice teacher should seek advice from the named practice educator, or link up with a teacher from the university or the student's personal tutor. They also include documenting student progress in appropriate sections of relevant documents, which may also have action-plan sections.

There are various ways in which the under-achieving students' learning can be facilitated to enable them to achieve their practice objectives in good time during the practice placement. Gopee (2008b) notes that such facilitation includes the following:

- Ensuring an initial interview is conducted by the named mentor during the first week of the placement identifying learning needs, and preferably formulating them into a learning contract.

- Observing closely the student's engagement in clinical interventions during the earlier part of the placement, but supervising them throughout the placement.
- Ensuring all key discussions, e.g. a mid-placement interview, incidents and meetings are documented.
- Compiling a realistic action plan to address areas of weakness, which of course does not have to wait till the mid-placement interview.
- Having full knowledge of, and ensuring you are following, the student's university's guidelines on mentoring.
- Accessing appropriate support for yourself as mentor, informally from colleagues and formally from established support mechanisms.
- Informing or involving practice education facilitators, a link teacher or a personal tutor of any unexpected student behaviour as soon as is appropriate.

In addition to the mid-placement review of competencies achieved, intermittent reviews should be conducted informally. Placements can occasionally be extended or repeated at a later point in time to enable the achievement of objectives. Furthermore, if the practice teacher feels competent in doing so, they can utilise their counselling skills to help a student. Cassidy (2009) reported on mentors themselves accessing the help of counsellors to clarify their own thinking in relation to 'under-achieving' students.

However, the practice teacher is accountable for pass or fail decisions for specific competencies. The consequence of a pass decision is that it is likely to increase the student's motivation to learn and achieve other competencies that can be achieved in the particular clinical setting. However, the practice teacher must award a fail for competencies for which the student does not present sufficient evidence of competence.

One of the consequences of failing to fail students is that later as a qualified healthcare professional they can unknowingly cause harm to patients or service users through 'commission or omissions', and through sub-standard practice or malpractice. Failing to fail students is thus itself unethical.

Documenting evidence of competence

Documenting students' progress based on evidence of achievement or non-achievement of practice competencies constitutes record-keeping. The NMC (2007a: 1) indicates that 'Record keeping is an integral part of nursing, midwifery and specialist community public health nursing practice. It is a tool of professional practice and one that should help the care process. It is not separate from this process and it is not an optional extra to be fitted in if circumstances allow'.

The NMC (2007a) and UK courts of law are quite clear about the importance and significance of effective record-keeping, and indicate that poor record-keeping is often a reflection of poor practice in other areas of the healthcare professional's work. The NMC (2009d) provides extensive guidelines on ways of ensuring effective record-keeping. The practice teacher documents nursing interventions as well as students' progress with the achievement of identified competencies, as well as with the management of under-achieving students.

Ethical competence in practice teaching

The principal aim of ensuring that a pass for the clinical skill is only awarded when there is sufficient evidence of competence on the part of the student for any particular competency is to ensure that they are fit for practice. Otherwise, as noted above, they can knowingly or unknowingly cause harm to patients and service users during clinical interventions, which in turn comprise unethical practice.

Ethics in healthcare is a well documented area. Thiroux and Krasemann (2007), for instance, indicate that the principles of ethical practice constitute valuing life, goodness and rightness, justice and fairness, truth telling and honesty, and individual freedom. The British Association for Counselling and Psychotherapy (2009) explains the principles of ethics a little differently by indicating that it comprises (i) fidelity (being trustworthy) (ii) autonomy, and (iii) beneficence (doing good), (iv) non-maleficence (doing no harm), (v) justice and (vi) self-respect.

Action point 6.2: Ethical practice in practice teaching

Our professional code of practice indicates that we must not do any harm to others, neither by commission nor omission. Make some notes on what you consider to be ethical practice teaching.

Healthcare professionals start to explore ethical practice very early in their careers, whereby they begin to develop their ethical competence. For instance, in the standards of proficiency for entry to the register, under 'Professional and ethical practice', the NMC (2004b: 26–7) indicates that a nurse must be competent to:

- practise in accordance with an ethical and legal framework which ensures the primacy of patient and client interest and wellbeing and respects confidentiality
- practise in a fair and anti-discriminatory way, acknowledging the differences in beliefs and cultural practices of individuals or groups.

Consequently, as a qualified healthcare professional, the practice teacher will already be competent in this component of professional practice, that is ethically competent, and should therefore be able to enable their students to develop ethical competence too. According to Sporrong et al. (2007), ethical competence is a psychological skill that comprises the ability of an individual to recognise, confront and analyse ethical situations, realise responsibilities and act in a way that is consistent with their professions' code of ethics. Codes of professional conduct, also referred to as 'good practice' (e.g. GMC (2006) *Good Medical Practice*) in some healthcare professions, are generally based on the ethics of the profession.

In relation to assessing students' clinical skills as well, practice teachers are acting ethically if the above principles, as well as the content of *The Code* (NMC, 2008d), are adhered to. Gopee (2008b) examined the current position with ethical practice related to assessing student nurses' clinical skills, and recommended that the ethical aspects of supporting learning and assessing student competence should be an explicit outcome of the educational preparation programmes for supporting learning (e.g. mentoring and practice teaching).

Conclusion

Chapter 6 focused on the practice teacher's responsibilities and accountability in the supervision of learning and in the assessment of specialist or advanced practice skills. It therefore explored the following areas of accountability:

- The reasons for analysing the practice teacher's accountability, what accountability is, the differences between accountability and responsibility as well as other related and inherent concepts; what we are accountable for and to whom; modes and dimensions of accountability; and the role of professional regulatory bodies.
- Specific responsibilities and areas of accountability of the practice teacher incorporating the accountability of safe and effective specialist or advanced practice for teaching and assessing specialist and advanced practice students, and signing off practice proficiency.
- Assessment and accountability, that is accountability for the decision to pass or fail students on specific competencies, ensuring the fitness for practice of specialist or advanced practice, ways of managing and supporting under-achieving students, cognisance of consequences of pass/fail decisions, and appropriate documentation of practice teacher activities.
- The ethical competence and implications of the practice teacher in the context of the facilitation of learning and in assessing clinical skills.

Practice teachers' responsibilities are partly self-determined and partly prescribed by their job descriptions. Accountability applies to all areas of the practice teacher role, such as caring for individuals when they are at their most vulnerable due to actual or threatened ill-health; and also towards students when they are endeavouring to achieve identified competencies. Although occasional lapses of professional conduct are reported, at most times, all healthcare professionals discharge their roles responsibly, and are prepared to account for the reasons for their clinical decisions.

The next chapter explores the reasons for the practice teacher having to exercise leadership. It countenances the reality of the quest for effective and efficient working in the face of the competing demands of clinical, teaching and administrative roles of the practice teacher, and consequently the ways in which the practice teacher fulfils this function, and also evaluates them.

7

Practice Teaching and Leadership

Introduction

In Chapter 6, the practice teacher's responsibilities and accountability in the supervision and assessment of learning were explored. Chapter 7 examines leadership, which is another dimension of the practice teacher's role, and encompasses definitions, theories and frameworks of leadership, and the application of these to practice teaching. The practice teacher exercises leadership as a specialist or advanced practitioner, and in the supervision of learning for pre-registration and post-qualifying students.

Chapter outcomes

On completion of this chapter you should be able to:

1 Explain the various reasons for, or the factors that are driving attention paid to, the leadership component of the practice teacher's role in the supervision of learning specialist and advanced practice skills.
2 Provide a critical account of what leadership means in the general context, including styles and theories of leadership, and frameworks that can also be utilised for leadership training and development.
3 Specify and justify the ways in which the practice teacher exercises leadership, and apply leadership theories to activities such as managing the competing demands of clinical practice, education and administrative roles of the practice teacher, and the application of knowledge and theory to practice.
4 Demonstrate an insight into how to lead education in clinical settings based on own expertise in creating and maintaining effective learning environments for students, utilising learning pathways based on patient journeys, and equality and diversity in education, as well as in an assessment of student competence.
5 Demonstrate a knowledge of evaluation, and critically analyse strategies for expertly evaluating the effectiveness of specialist and advanced practice, and of the teaching, learning and assessment experiences of healthcare profession students.

Why leadership in practice teaching?

There are several reasons for practice teachers having to be aware of their leadership functions and responsibilities. One reason is that as specialist or advanced practitioners, and therefore experts in clinical interventions in their field of practice, practice teachers have to lead by example, and another is that leadership is consistently highlighted as an attribute and function of CNSs, ANPs and similar roles. Both the Scottish Government (2008) and Humphreys et al. (2007), for instance, identify the four key functions of senior clinicians as expert practice, leadership, education and research.

In general, nurses are in a better position to take the lead in several areas of clinical activities, that is they can suggest decisions, solutions to problematic situations, and so on, as they have a fuller knowledge of all eventualities in the clinical setting by their mere presence in that setting 24 hours a day. Moreover, Cunningham and Kitson (2000), Kouzes and Posner (2007) and others suggest that all nurses may be in a position to take the lead in some way, and that there is no evidence that leadership qualities are in-born or inherited, but can be developed through appropriate educational programmes.

Furthermore, on exploring the research literature on leadership, Alimo-Metcalfe (1996) observes that the satisfaction that staff achieve from their work is in part determined by the style of leadership they work under, and that leadership style and organisational culture are associated with an increase in productivity. Huczynski and Buchanan (2007) suggest that leadership is a critical determinant of organisational effectiveness, and that it is associated with positions of power, influence and status.

In healthcare, Manley (1997) indicates that there is a correlation between effective nursing leadership and the quality of patient care experienced by patients, and it also facilitates staff empowerment and practice development. For an evaluation of the effectiveness of leadership in clinical settings, a RCN-sponsored study conducted by King's College-based researchers concluded that there is a range of critical factors related particularly to nurse leadership; one is related to a reduction in patient infection rates and, more widely, to quality patient care and clinical outcomes (Griffiths et al., 2008).

Leadership is also one of the eight domains of learning and assessment in practice identified by the NMC (2008a), and its overall descriptor states that the practice teacher must 'Demonstrate leadership skills for education within practice and academic settings' (p. 58).

Action point 7.1 – Why leadership in practice teaching?

Consider and make notes on why you think the NMC indicates that leadership is an important inherent component of the practice teacher role.

The outcomes for a practice teacher under the leadership domain are to:

- provide practice leadership and expertise in the application of knowledge and skills based on evidence
- demonstrate the ability to lead education in practice, working across practice and academic settings

- manage competing demands of practice and education related to supporting different practice levels of students
- lead and contribute to an evaluation of the effectiveness of learning and assessment in practice.

The first outcome refers to the practice teacher's expertise in applying evidence-based knowledge to practice. This concept does not only signify effective practice that is evidence-based (as discussed in Chapter 4), but also how the practice teacher is explicitly being a role model of best practice, as an exemplary leader providing transformational leadership, as do, for example, modern matrons and consultant nurses.

The third outcome recognises that there are competing demands in the practice teacher's working hours. This situation has been highlighted for some time, and formed a key finding of the landmark study by Phillips et al. (2000), but also later by Nettleton and Bray (2008). Because the practice teacher recognises such demands on their time, they consequently have to plan even further ahead, and prioritise their clinical activities to ensure that their practice teaching role is also fully accommodated.

Another reason for exploring the practice teacher's leadership is that all nurses' day-to-day activities include their management functions, and according to Mintzberg's (1990) study the ten roles of the manager include being a leader, with the other roles being a figurehead, liaison, monitor, entrepreneur, and so on.

The *High Quality Care for All* (DH, 2008b) report recommends the setting up of the NHS Leadership Council which will have a particular focus on standards, and with a dedicated budget will be able to commission leadership development programmes. The definition of leadership implied in the report and used to guide these recommendations includes:

- posts with significant leadership requirement should be filled with strong leadership potentials
- behaviours and values enacted by those who fill leadership posts should create a culture of leadership which supports quality improvement throughout the system
- career development for all those with the potential to fill leadership positions
- development programmes and a broader infrastructure, which identify, develop and support people to fill leadership posts throughout the system

What is leadership? Definitions and scope of the concept

A quick tour of the concept of leadership reveals that it comprises:

- several definitions of leadership, which reveal a common theme running through them
- an overlap between functions, roles, and the behaviours of leaders and managers
- styles of leadership based on personality traits
- theories of effective leadership
- frameworks of leadership capabilities that the individual can develop through leadership development programmes, which benefit patient or service-user care and teamwork directly.

All five components have significance for specialist and advanced practitioners in their practice teacher role, even if they are not in appointed management positions. With regard to definitions, Gopee and Galloway (2009: 48) define leadership in the context of clinical manager's roles as comprising 'the ability to motivate, inspire and energise individuals and groups to identify and achieve healthcare goals'. Sullivan and Decker (2009: 45) indicate that 'A leader is anyone who uses interpersonal skills to influence others to accomplish a specific goal'. On the other hand, Huczynski and Buchanan (2007) indicate that leadership is a related concept that refers to the process of influencing the activities of an organised group in its efforts towards goal-setting and goal achievement. Mullins (2007: 363) suggests that leadership is 'a relationship through which one person influences the behaviour or actions of other people'.

All these current definitions of leadership have a common theme running through them, which is that leaders influence the behaviour and thinking of their followers. The leader exerts influence in various ways such as by having the most acceptable visions for the group, by 'leading by example', and so on.

Action point 7.2 – What do I already know about leaders and leadership?

Based on your experience of leaders and managers in healthcare settings, complete the following sentences:

The healthcare professionals who are leaders in my workplace are ....

The differences between leaders and managers are ....

The activities and behaviours of a 'good leader' are ....

The activities and behaviours of a 'poor leader' are ....

Nurse leaders are visible in healthcare settings as senior staff nurses, team leaders, modern matrons, nurse consultants, and so on. In thinking about the third and fourth items in Action Point 7.2, you might have been wondering how helpful such subjective thoughts can be to the practice teacher role. In fact you will note shortly that many of your responses are reflected in both previous and current research findings, which consequently can be utilised as frameworks for leadership capability self-assessment and development programmes.

Styles and theories of effective leadership

Leaders become known for the styles of leadership they display, which are based on personality traits. They might demonstrate leadership using:

- an autocratic style
- a participative/democratic style
- a laissez-faire style
- a bureaucratic style
- a political style.

Parish (2006) reports on a study by management consultants that compared high-performing ward managers with those who showed lower levels of performance. In their findings they identify six styles of leadership:

- *Directive* – to achieve immediate compliance.
- *Visionary* – to provide long-term direction and vision.
- *Affiliative* – to create harmony.
- *Participative* – to build on commitment and generate new ideas.
- *Pace-setting* – to accomplish tasks to a high standard.
- *Coaching* – to develop others in the long term.

Goleman's (2000) study revealed that the most effective leaders tend to combine different styles of leadership for different situations as necessary.

There are several theories of leadership that have evolved from research over time. Box 7.1 identifies the main ones that practice teachers can draw on.

Box 7.1   Theories of leadership

Trait theories | • Personal attributes of leaders
Functional theories | • Functions of leadership position
| • Action-centred leadership
Contemporary theories | • Transactional leadership
| • Transformational leadership
| • Connective leadership
| • Servant leadership

Trait theories refer to the personal qualities of individuals in leadership positions, which include self-confidence, persuasiveness, charm, personal power, extraordinary ideas and strong (often unconventional) convictions. Current research on leadership, for example Kouzes and Posner (2007), tends to identify specific personality traits or characteristics of leaders. Following their global survey of specific personality traits of the most successful leaders, Kouzes and Posner identify the qualities of 'admired leaders' as honest, forward looking, competent and inspiring (in order of most significant qualities first). Other traits rated as significant are: intelligent, fair-minded, broad-minded, supportive, straightforward, dependable, co-operative, determined, imaginative, ambitious, courageous, caring, mature, loyal, self-controlled, independent (also in order of preference). On nursing leadership, research includes a study by Cook and Leathard (2004) which identifies the key attributes of effective leaders and 'facilitative factors'.

The activities of leaders, on the other hand, fall under functional leadership theories, which as the term implies, refer to the functions of leadership. Kouzes and Posner's (2007) study also identifies the 'practices' (i.e. activities) of 'exemplary leaders'. One of the most prominent functional theories of leadership is Adair's (1988) action-centred leadership, which signifies that effective leaders address three sets of needs within the organisation. These are task needs, individual needs and team- or group-maintenance needs, which the functional leader must ensure are met.

Under contemporary leadership theories, currently the most documented are transactional leadership, transformational leadership, connective leadership and servant leadership. Transactional leadership refers to leaders whose main focus is on maintaining an equilibrium by working fully in accordance with policies and procedures. Transformational leaders tend to refer to individuals who effect radical or revolutionary changes by merging the goals, desires and values of their followers with their own, stimulate growth and development, and discourage dependence. A comparison of transformational and transactional theories is presented in Table 7.1

Table 7.1   *Comparison of transformational and transactional leadership approaches*

Transformational leadership	Transactional leadership
The leader succeeds in merging their own goals, desires and values with those of followers and the organisation into a common goal	The leader aims to maintain the smooth functioning of the work setting
Employees develop a commitment to the group's/organisation's vision	Tends to ensure the tasks to be performed are the highest priority
Instils a belief in followers that they have the capability to achieve group and individual goals	Ensures policies and procedures are strictly adhered to
Discourages dependence and stimulates growth and development	Tends to be strategically focused, with short- or medium-term organisational goals
Challenges subordinates views in order to enable them to explore concepts in depth and detail	Believes in, and fosters, coaching and sheltered learning
Always ready to positively reinforce strengths and achievements, informally and personally	Uses material rewards when reinforcing achievements
Is passionate about existing and new ventures	Has self-interest high on the agenda
Does not separate work life from home life completely	Treats home and work as separate areas of their life

Research on these two types of leadership includes Lipley's (2004) work, which found that a mix of transformational leadership and transactional leadership is better that the laissez-faire approach at making staff more enthusiastic about their jobs. Clegg (2000) found that transformational leadership has positive effects on team performance and the quality of patient care in a community trust.

Connective leadership refers to the theory that the leader fosters collaborative intra-organisational and inter-organisational relationships – for example between clinical settings in the same specialism. Servant leadership does not comprise a set of techniques or guidelines to improve productivity, but is based more on the leader's underpinning attitude and beliefs about the people they lead, with the aim to 'serve' them, that act with their interests at heart. It is therefore based on the premise that leadership implies a desire to serve.

Framework of leadership capabilities

As leadership is increasingly perceived as comprising specific skills that training can develop, there are various leadership skills training programmes that are available, some as short courses, others as diploma or degree courses. The RCN's

(Large et al., 2005) 12-month Clinical Leadership Programme for the professional development of clinical leaders is one of them. Kouzes and Posner's (2007) 'practices of exemplary leadership', which can also be used for the self-assessment of own leadership activities and capabilities, and subsequent self-development, are as follows:

- *Model the way*
  1. Find your voice by clarifying your personal values
  2. Set examples by aligning actions with shared values
- *Inspire a shared vision*
  3. Envision the future by imagining exciting and ennobling possibilities
  4. Enlist others in a common vision by appealing to shared aspirations
- *Challenge the process*
  5. Search for opportunities by seeking innovative ways to change, grow and improve.
  6. Experiment and take risks by constantly generating small wins and learn from mistakes
- *Enable others to act*
  7. Foster collaboration by promoting co-operative goals and building trust
  8. Strengthen others by sharing power and discretion
- *Encourage the heart*
  9. Recognise contributions by showing appreciation for individual excellence
  10. Celebrate the values and victories by creating a spirit of community.

The practice teacher's leadership in clinical practice

Research by Kouzes and Posner (2007) identifies the activities that individuals in leadership positions need to engage in to be effective leaders. These activities can also be applied to their practice teaching role. '*Enable others to act*', for example, is an area that directly relates to the practice teacher enabling their students to provide care independently, that is they are given the responsibility to perform clinical interventions without close supervision when they are deemed competent to do so. Other similar reports were identified in Chapter 1. For the component '*Model the way*' the practice teacher can exercise leadership by being a role model in all areas of the NMC's domains and outcomes for practice teachers.

Challenges in supporting learning

Kouzes and Posner's (2007) category '*Challenge the process*' is at the heart of activities that practice teachers engage in, in that the current contexts in which the practice teacher operates are wide and varied. It involves managing the competing demands of clinical practice (third NMC outcome under leadership domain, noted earlier in this chapter), teaching and education, and the administrative roles of a practice teacher, which therefore require adequate advanced planning, whilst taking several factors into account, such as ensuring their leadership is reflected in creating and maintaining a learning environment in the practice setting, educating across practice and academic settings, the integration of theory and practice, equality and diversity in clinical learning, and assessing competence, and ensuring the fitness for practice of specialist or advanced practitioners.

Proactive planning and time management are therefore central to the practice teacher role, and so competence in the above-mentioned areas is essential. The practice teacher has to have expertise and must lead in these areas, whilst also taking into account the current context of healthcare delivery, political, economic, social expectations, and so on. To support this function, some form of mentorship is recommended in addition to supervision and clinical supervision for senior nurses (including practice teachers) as they are among those who are very likely to be in a position of leadership (Frankel, 2008). Frankel suggests five to 30 minutes of structured mentorship time during each shift, which is dedicated to a discussion on their leadership. The content of this mentoring can form the basis for reflection-on-action by the senior nurse. The characteristics of an effective leader can be determined and agreed on beforehand.

Transformational leadership in practice teaching

'*Inspire a shared vision*' (Kouzes and Posner, 2007) is an area that practice teachers as specialist or advanced practitioners tend to address quite well. Literature, in particular research publications, on how the practice teacher exercises leadership is sparse, but there is an abundance of publications demonstrating how they can implement their vision for patient or service-user care as specialist and advanced practitioners. In particular there are several examples of nurse-led healthcare provision.

For instance, Blakemore (2008) reports on how the implementation of a new skin care regimen for patients at risk of developing pressure ulcers reduced significantly the incidence of pressure sores. The effectiveness of nurse-led services for patients with diabetes reported in *Nursing Standard News* (2008c) is another example, as is the case for specialist rheumatoid arthritis services reported by Ryan (2008). Raftery et al. (2005), researchers in Birmingham and Aberdeen, jointly explored the impact of nurse-led clinics in the promotion of medical and lifestyle components of secondary prevention (of coronary heart disease), and reported that they are effective in terms of life years saved, and also cost effective.

McIntosh and Tolson (2009) reported on leadership as a component of the nurse-consultant role, in which they evaluated the activities of nurse consultants (in Scotland), predominantly in relation to the attributes of transformational leadership, which they based on semi-structured interviews with nurse consultants and other 'stakeholders' who worked with them. They found that nurse consultants do use approaches that approximate the features of transformational leadership, such as developing a vision for the service, acting as mediators and champions, and exerting control over complex change initiatives. Techniques of leadership included managing change, assertion, interpersonal skills and intellectual effort in achieving outcomes, and taking risks. These posts require appropriate support if they are to be sustainable.

Xiao (2008) explored nurse educators' leadership behaviours in implementing mandatory continuing nursing education in China, and found that proactive-type educators share the core attributes of transformational leaders and are able to enable mandatory continuing nursing education, while reactive-type educators show the attributes of transactional leaders.

Mockett et al. (2006) reported on the strategies used by clinical education leaders to manage change from non-aligned, ad hoc, unsystematic practices (in continuing education provision) to one based on accountability, professionalism and evidence-based education. The latter methods were implemented using a systematic change management framework, which was also evaluated using Kirkpatrick's (2005) model of evaluation (discussed later in this chapter). The success of this effective change is attributed to 'strong leadership, perseverance and understanding of the organisation's culture' (p. 409).

Leadership in theory–practice integration

In the context of 'Challenge the process' (Kouzes and Posner, 2007) another area of leadership is in theory–practice integration. Predominantly because there is a limit to the resources (time, equipment, materials and money) that are available for care delivery, at times clinical interventions are not performed exactly in the way the theory indicates they should be performed, albeit they still constitute safe and effective practice.

Until recently, there have been debates in nursing on the notion of a theory–practice gap (e.g. Ousey and Gallagher, 2007). Lately, predominantly initiated by nursing statutory bodies, the concept has shifted to theory–practice integration. The theory–practice relationship refers to performing specific clinical interventions through the healthcare trust's identified procedures and clinical guidelines, or good practice guidelines, but the concept of a theory–practice gap suggests that these procedures and protocols are not being followed in the practice setting. Consequently, it is suggested that instead of focusing on a 'gap', the clinically based teacher should clearly inform their learners how and how far they are following the guidelines, and which components they are adapting to the specific circumstances, based on an in-built flexibility in the guideline. Senior practitioners such as specialist and advanced practitioners tend to have some scope for adapting guidelines, based on their professional expertise and experience.

Audits provide one means of monitoring the extent to which theory and practice are integrated, and to identify if there is any gap in this, and research is an alternative means. Lankshear et al. (2008) reported on a study that found that patient safety alerts, which constitute procedures for reporting, avoiding repeating and learning from potentially dangerous mistakes, are not routinely implemented. This situation is an example of the constitution of a theory that is not applied in practice consistently, thereby creating a theory–practice gap. In this instance, the reasons for not implementing the procedure related to the day-to-day material use of nasogastric tubes and Guedal airways and were identified as staff not fully understanding the procedure, and the trust dismissing aspects of these alerts as irrelevant.

However, another reason for this so-called gap may be that the theory was not derived from empirical studies, nor was it tested rigorously prior to implementation. It could also have been constituted through a group opinion of selected experts, as a number of procedures are.

There are a number of reasons for difficulties in applying theory to healthcare settings and to patient care. Typically, theories on how to perform clinical interventions are taught in classroom settings, and practice is how they are actually

... the clinical setting. When a 'theory–practice gap' was identified as ... issue several decades ago, the actions taken to resolve the problem included new roles such as clinical teachers, joint appointments and lecturers–practitioners. However, all these roles have proved problematic. Some of the ways in which theory and practice are integrated include:

- by university teachers ensuring clinical skills are taught based on national guidelines and procedures, and that changes are communicated to mentors and practice teachers, through practice education facilitators, for instance
- reflective practice, and reflective recordings in personal journals
- trust-based practitioners attending trust-based updates on a wider range of clinical interventions
- clinical skill updates that provide opportunities for practising the skill under supervision, both at the update session, and subsequently
- when teaching theories related to clinical interventions, there must be full opportunities for discussion on their application to clinical settings.

The practice teacher thus needs to remain aware that in their role in theory–practice integration, certain theories might not be founded on a firm enough basis, and therefore has to remain open minded about them, and see questioning theory–practice relationship as a healthy learning opportunity. This is despite being duty bound to implement procedures set by their employer.

Competing demands of practice and education, and forward planning

A practice teacher is a specialist or advanced practitioner, will have a teaching role and might even have managerial or organisational responsibilities, as required, and needs to manage the competing demands of practice and education, signing off practice proficiency, and equality and diversity in education. The first two components may include teaching patients or service users how to restore and maintain their health as much as possible. All such activities require quality time and considered proactive forward planning.

The practice teacher might encounter the competing demands of clinical practice, education, administrative duties and self-updating activities fairly frequently. Various studies such as that by Philips et al. (2000) found that the clinician in the teaching role, for example that of mentor, often struggles with the competing demands of practice and education. These include being pulled in different directions because of specialist or advanced practice duties, in addition to their teaching and assessing roles during practice placements. Other more recent studies still highlight similar problems in this area (e.g. Nettleton and Bray, 2008) (discussed in Chapter 8).

The practice teacher's leadership in educating and assessing students

Creating and maintaining an optimum learning environment

As noted in Chapter 3, the practice teacher's roles include input into ensuring that their clinical setting functions as an effective learning environment. As autonomous

professionals, practice teachers must manifest leadership in this
ey need to, but generally this comprises a team effort at local
a learning environment is created and maintained by teams on the
primary healthcare centre, but also at an organisational level. At both
rning ethos needs to prevail informally first and then be implemented
ally.

NMC identifies the practice teacher's role in creating and maintaining the
actice setting as a learning environment under the domains 'creating an environment for learning' and 'leadership'. Based on previous research, the NMC (2008a)
requires practice teachers and other education facilitators to be competent in these
domains in order to enhance and maximise students' learning.

A learning environment can be sustained informally by ensuring a learning culture
prevails. Gopee (2008a: 88) defines a learning environment as follows: '. . . a clinical
setting that constitutes a learning environment comprises a psychosocial ethos and
culture with related supportive resources that foster mutual learning amongst all
stakeholder healthcare professionals, learners and clientele, and where care and
treatment are founded on evidence-based practice'. It is particularly significant to note
that the learning environment requires a 'psychosocial ethos and culture', which
comprises the informal dimension of sustaining a learning ethos. The definition also
suggests a need for the necessary learning 'resources', which require a more systematic
approach that can enable learning throughout the organisation, that is at healthcare-
trust or unit level, whereupon a budget is regularly allocated for designated learning
facilities such as a dedicated teaching and learning area in the clinical setting,
information technology facilities, and so on.

Another systematic dimension is through an annual educational audit of each clinical
setting, where healthcare profession students are allocated to practice placements.
Education audit forms are jointly and carefully designed by the university and
associated healthcare trusts to ensure the criteria for suitable learning environments are
informed, that is based on research findings and on national guidelines and policies.
The audit is performed annually to ascertain each setting's suitability for student
placement, and is documented appropriately as it is also an NMC (2004b) requirement.

Various publications and research contribute to identifying the criteria for
effective learning environments through education audits. In *Placement in Focus*,
the DH/ENB (2001), for instance, lists several criteria that practice settings have
to institute to be considered an effective learning environment. They are
presented under four key headings:

1   Providing practice placements.
2   Practice learning environment.
3   Student support.
4   Assessment of practice.

The RCN's (2002) advice to students in relation to what is an effective learning
environment in practice settings includes:

- the practice placement has a favourable culture for learning
- students have the opportunity to experience 24-hour, seven days a week care at
  some stage in the placement programme

- students are encouraged to question practices that they feel are unsafe or not research based
- students are helped to feel part of the team
- staff practise care in line with the philosophy of the environment
- there is evidence of multi-professional team working within the documentation of care
- there is effective interpersonal communication between team members
- notice and topic boards are used to good effect, with relevant information to help students
- learning resources are available for students to use – for example, current books and journals, research materials, information technology and on-line resources.

Following on from the RCN's recommendations related to learning resources, naturally the staff who are normally employed in the particular clinical setting also comprise a useful learning resource. There should not only be adequate numbers of permanent staff who should be able to facilitate learning and who are accessible, but they should also be content and satisfied with their work conditions. An appropriate work environment such as those in Magnet Hospitals in the USA would be a precondition for an effective learning environment.

Action point 7.3 – The clinical setting as a learning environment

Unless you have done so recently, explore with a colleague in your clinical setting, or as a team, all the actions that are taken by you to ensure the setting has an effective learning environment. Find out also when the most recent education audit was conducted, and what the outcomes were.

Clinical settings that are utilised as practice placements include primary care settings, but there is a dearth of research specifically related to these settings as learning environments. Lofmark et al. (2008) suggest a model of supervision of learning during practice placements, which they derive from existing theories and empirical studies, and which is made up of four components: a head supervisor, two named mentors for the day-to-day supervision of learning, access to patient care, and the presentation of a seminar demonstrating the integration of theory and practice. The authors report that the model is effective, but they also indicate that there is an insufficient application of research to nursing care, and insufficient planned time for reflection.

Although the achievement of specific clinical competencies may be a course requirement during practice placements, another key activity that the practice teacher has to undertake is to enable the student to integrate theory and practice, and to apply theories and principles of learning to their teaching. Placement learning can thus incorporate skills teaching followed by a reference to the underlying theory, which is the pragmatic style of learning. It can incorporate reflective practice based on Kolb's (1984) theory of learning.

Learning during placements largely includes planned learning opportunities, but also capitalises on incidental learning opportunities. Another systematic dimension that contributes to a learning environment is the utilisation of learning pathways for students, which are based on patients' journeys through healthcare, which itself incorporates inter-professional input into learning, and therefore also inter-professional learning.

Patients' journeys and learning pathways

The facilitation of learning can take place in different clinical settings, for example primary care, advanced emergency care, palliative care, or in caring for patients with long-term conditions. A fuller picture of the patient's illness, and progress with it, can be identified by ascertaining the 'patient's journey' through the healthcare system. Patient journeys can form the basis for designing learning pathways for students, which can provide even more structure to student learning, as well as make learning interactive.

Utilising learning pathways based on patient journeys is gradually establishing a firm hold in professional learning especially as part of inter-professional learning in pre- and post-registration programmes. There tends to be a module in the first semester of pre-registration education, which addresses IPE in facilitated sessions, some face-to-face and others online, to enable students to engage with, explore and identify ways of approaching inter-professional learning. They soon tend to appreciate the benefits of inter-professional learning, and work out ways of ensuring this occurs.

Often a case study is presented to a multi-disciplinary group of students, and from their current knowledge of the provisions in their profession they suggest ways in which the patient can be helped to regain their health. Both face-to-face and on-line engagements present a healthy approach to learning about the well co-ordinated delivery of care and treatment.

Using the 'hub and spokes model' in planning practice placements for specialist practice students, the practice teacher needs to incorporate inter-professional learning in the schedule as it brings a range of benefits to all – healthcare staff, patients and their relatives.

Equality and diversity in education

The practice teacher's leadership includes addressing ways of meeting equality and diversity policies in education. Policies and laws on equality and diversity play a very important role in enabling healthcare organisations to meet the individual learning needs of healthcare professionals and students with disabilities. Laws such as the Disability Discrimination Act (1995) (and the 2004 amendments), and the Special Educational Needs and Disability Act (2001) indicate the actions that supervisors should take to assist individuals with disabilities.

The Disability Discrimination Act (1995) states that it is unlawful to discriminate against a disabled person in the field of employment and requires the employer to make reasonable adjustments if employment arrangements place disabled people at a substantial disadvantage. Its 2004 amendment brought practical work experience placements within the scope of the Disability Discrimination Act and regulatory bodies such as the NMC.

However, the Disability Rights Commission Report (2007), which resulted from a year-long investigation into disabled people's access to the professions of teaching, nursing and social work, revealed that there is:

- still a stigma attached to disabilities and individuals resist disclosing their disability to employers
- still confusion on what actually constitutes a disability
- a lack of active promotion of the entry of disabled people into the professions
- a need for greater dialogue between occupational health services and HEIs
- a need for greater guidance into what constitutes a reasonable adjustment.

White (2007) researched the nature of the support nursing students with dyslexia receive and require in healthcare settings during practice placements, aiming to determine whether pre-registration nursing students with dyslexia experience specific problems in developing clinical competence, identify the strategies that they use and how they may be supported in clinical practice. The study revealed that students' difficulties in clinical practice fell into three categories: dealing with information; performing the role; and administering drugs. Specific supporting measures tailored to meet their specific needs include: informal and formal support networks; portable information technology equipment; and personal strategies for rehearsing difficult tasks, such as the handover report.

Guidance on ways of ensuring equality and diversity requirements are met is provided by several organisations, including the RCN (2007c) and locally by healthcare employers and universities.

Leadership in the assessment of clinical competence

Leadership implies being one step ahead of followers. It signifies having an insight into what needs to be done, including what recipients of the service expect, and planning ahead so that these expectations can be met. How the practice teacher achieves this with regard to the facilitation of learning was discussed in the preceding section.

As to how the practice teacher meets expectations related to the assessment of competence, this also requires forward planning, which can be achieved by having substantial or full insight into the student's expectations well before they arrive on a placement. This can be followed by having a plan or at least a blueprint of clinical experiences that can facilitate the achievement of placement competencies. Such planning is vitally important as it improves the efficiency of the service, and also because recent research (e.g. Nettleton and Bray, 2008) identified how supervisors of learning struggle to make time for their students.

Leadership in evaluating the effectiveness of practice teaching

The practice teacher must evaluate the effectiveness of practice teaching and assessment within a variety of clinical settings which their named students will experience during practice placements. Evaluation of the effectiveness of teaching, learning and assessment, including those in academic settings, reflects the efficacy and quality of the programme. Evaluation, as a concept in its own right, is different from research and assessment, although there are common elements within them.

Action point 7.4 – What is evaluation?

Constitute your own definition of the term 'evaluation', in the context of evaluating the facilitation of student learning in healthcare settings.

There are distinctions between the overlapping terms evaluation, monitoring, assessment, research and validation as they all refer to obtaining recipients' views on the provision, but the terms also signify other different activities. Evaluation, in the context of practice teaching, signifies inviting and obtaining comments from students (and possibly peers) on the strengths of their teaching and areas suggested for improvement.

With regard to exactly what it is that practice teachers evaluate, they will evaluate all components of their role, namely in:

- patient or service user care to ensure they are safe and effective
- teaching and assessing students
- management and leadership
- evidence-based practice and research implementation.

There are various types of evaluation, including:

- public evaluation – private/self-evaluation
- external (to the healthcare trust/unit) evaluation – internal evaluation
- continuous evaluation – episodic/intermittent evaluation
- formative – summative or final evaluation
- case-specific evaluation – generalised or holistic evaluation
- quantitative or qualitative evaluation.

Reasons for evaluating and monitoring
the quality of teaching, learning and assessment

There are several reasons for evaluating any educational activity. One reason is that the dictionary definition of the word evaluation itself means determining the value or worth of the item being evaluated. We evaluate care and treatment to determine their effectiveness, and as such it is one of the four components of the nursing process itself (the other three being assessment, planning and implementation).

Action point 7.5 – Evaluating practice teaching

Preferably in discussion with a peer, consider and make notes on the following questions.

1 What are the various reasons for practice teachers needing to evaluate their work activities?
2 Specifically, what does the practice teacher evaluate?

If you have had the opportunity to discuss the above questions with a peer, or within your own thinking, you would have come up with a few reasons for evaluation practice teaching. You might have decided that questions (1) and (2) are closely linked, and for question (2), you might have felt that the practice teacher needs to evaluate all the components of their clinical activities, namely hands-on clinical interventions, as well as the way they manage and organise care, and is aware of research and practice development on their area of practice, as well as teaching, learning and assessment activities. These areas might form part of the key areas in your job description, but alternatively such components are also identifiable as core dimensions of the *NHS KSF* (DH, 2004a) noted in Chapter 1. Thus technically it is possible to evaluate all the activities that the practice teacher engages in, in their day-to-day worth activities, and is therefore accountable for.

Another reason for an evaluation of practice teaching is that under the domain evaluation of learning, the NMC (2008a: 54) indicates that the practice teacher must 'Determine strategies for evaluating learning in practice and academic settings to ensure that the NMC standards of proficiency for registration or recording a qualification at a level above initial registration have been met'. The outcomes for this standard are:

- designing evaluation strategies to determine the effectiveness of practice and academic experience accessed by students at both registration level and those in education at a level beyond initial registration
- collaborating with other members of the teaching team to judge and develop learning, assessment and support appropriate to practice and levels of education
- collecting evidence on the quality of education in practice, and determining how well NMC requirements for standards of proficiency are being achieved.

Other reasons for evaluating include:

- to identify areas of practice teaching activities that can be improved
- to enhance performance
- to gauge whether students' learning is pitched at the appropriate level
- continuing self-assessment of competence in professional practice as a requirement of employment
- to ascertain whether the intended effects of interventions are being achieved
- because it is a component of the healthcare setting's quality assurance mechanism
- because it is professional 'good practice'
- because it is a form of empirical investigation, through data collection.

Based on the above comments on why we should evaluate, it becomes obvious that evaluation forms part of the process of quality monitoring and enhancement.

Monitoring the quality of professional education

There are a number of ways in which the quality of education delivered in HEIs is monitored, one of the principal aims of which is to ensure that they are fit for purpose, practice and award, as identified in the Dearing Report (NCIHE, 1997) and by the NMC (2004b). The processes by which courses are planned and approved were discussed in Chapter 3. All higher-education programmes are quality assessed by the QAA, and healthcare profession programmes are monitored by the NMC through an organisation known as Mott MacDonald.

The quality of healthcare profession education is also regularly monitored by several other agencies, for example the local Strategic Health Authority, the Skills for Health (2009b) (as noted in Chapter 5), and others. Each organisation has its own framework and criteria for ascertaining the quality of education provision.

Each of these monitoring organisations requires detailed information on how the quality of programmes are monitored internally, that is through the university's own quality assurance mechanisms, and on the day of the monitoring visit they ask further questions based on their own checklists of criteria which are generally made available before the visit. Internal quality assurance mechanisms include an evaluation of all components of education provision. Furthermore, stakeholders, that is the purchasing healthcare trusts, also regularly monitor and receive evaluations of educational programmes.

Evaluation of the effectiveness of practice teaching and assessment

For the teaching and learning provision for SPQ and ANP students during a practice placement, practice teachers should conduct their own evaluation of these experiences by seeking feedback from students, especially at the end of the placement. They can seek to ascertain the useful experiences, as well as aspects of the placement that can be improved.

The evaluations can be written or verbal, and the former can be structured by utilising an established framework.

Action point 7.6 – How do you evaluate the teaching and learning you provide to your students?

Consider the competences and each outcome for practice teachers under 'Evaluation of learning', and identify exactly how you can apply them to practice teaching in your clinical setting.

In the evaluation of activities in social sciences, both quantitative and qualitative data need to be obtained for a fuller view of recipients' perceptions of the provision. Evaluation of teaching, learning and assessing in practice settings can be undertaken formally and informally in a number of ways – Box 7.2 identifies a number of these mechanisms.

Box 7.2   Mechanisms for evaluating learning during practice placements

- Using evaluation form(s)
- Verbal feedback – requested/ volunteered
- Using questionnaire(s)
- Continuous monitoring of student's clinical competence
- Observing the student's motivation to learn

- Verbal questions and answers
- Observing clinical skill performance – directly and indirectly
- Checking whether objectives are being met
- Reflective account
- Consultation with colleagues
- Quiz – on paper/verbal
- Discussing competencies booklet
- Observing how other teachers teach the skill
- Self-evaluation
- Asking the student to teach others, e.g. patients and junior staff, and observe them
- Feedback from the university through link teachers, PEFs, etc.
- Active participation in course planning for shorter clinical courses, control, etc.

The content of practice placement experience and learning evaluation forms should reflect components that comprise an effective clinical learning environment, such as whether:

- students are given an orientation to the practice setting, including where practice procedures and clinical guidelines are located
- learning needs are identified as early as possible for the placement area
- mentor support
- continuous feedback on performance of clinical interventions
- informed when clinical competencies were being assessed.

The form would include blank spaces for further comments, namely qualitative data. Furthermore, various models and frameworks for evaluation are available for the practice teacher to choose from and utilise. One of the most effective frameworks for evaluating healthcare professionals' clinical activities systematically is the Donabedian (1988) model which comprises evaluating the structures (i.e. the resources required such as equipment, building, staff, materials required to deliver the service); process (the procedure, protocols, staff training, etc. required); and the outcome (i.e. achievement of the intended outcomes). This can be seen from another angle as structure evaluation, process evaluation and outcome evaluation. Better practices can be implemented at individual level, team level, organisational and even at national and international levels, and need to be evaluated at the appropriate level.

Alternatively, Kirkpatrick and Kirkpatrick's (2005) model of evaluation, which comprises four levels of evaluation, should prove useful:

Reaction (level 1): how participants have reacted to the programme.
Learning (level 2): what participants have learnt from the programme in line with programme objectives such as an increase in skill or knowledge, or a change of attitude that can be applied to practice settings.
Behaviour (level 3): whether what was learnt is being applied on the job, the extent to which a change in personal behaviour has occurred, as a result of the programme.
Results (level 4): whether that application is achieving results – tangible and intangible results.

The practice teacher can utilise either of these frameworks to evaluate a facilitation of learning and an assessment of competence activities; that is learning and assessment can be evaluated by examining the structures, processes and outcomes at individual, team and organisational levels (Donabedian model), or by examining reaction, behaviour, learning and results (Kirkpatrick model) as suggested herewith.

Level	Criteria
Reaction	
Learning	
Behaviour	
Results (quantitative and qualitative)	

Both Donabedian's and Kirkpatrick's models of evaluation are tested and proven frameworks for the evaluation of teaching activities. Logically, following an evaluation, action has to be taken to maintain areas of good practice, rectify weaknesses, and explore the potentials of suggestions for improvement.

Conclusion

In this chapter, how the practice teacher exercises leadership was analysed, which is an activity that encompasses the advanced planning of a facilitation of learning for facilitating learning and an assessment of competence to ensure a fitness for practice in specialist and advanced clinical practice. It incorporates managing the competing demands of clinical, teaching and administrative roles, time management, and the integration of theory and practice. The chapter therefore addressed:

- Why there is leadership in practice teaching, and what leadership is itself, and included definitions and the scope of the concept of leadership, theories of effective leadership and frameworks for developing leadership capabilities.
- The practice teacher's leadership in clinical practice, in dealing with the challenges encountered in supporting learning, in theory–practice integration, in managing the competing demands of practice and education, and in forward planning.

- The practice teacher's leadership in educating and assessing students, in creating and maintaining an optimum learning environment, utilising learning pathways, ensuring equality and diversity in education, and leadership in the assessment of clinical competence.
- Leading the monitoring of teaching, learning and the assessment of specialist or advanced practice, evaluating the effectiveness and quality of practice teaching and assessment, including the reasons for evaluating in both practice and academic settings, and utilising recognised frameworks and models of evaluation.

Based on the areas of clinical and teaching activities that practice teachers encounter, exercising leadership emerges as an essential key component of the role. Chapter 8 will examine the issues and contemporary further developments in practice teaching in the healthcare and social-care professions.

8

Issues and Further Developments in Facilitating the Acquisition of Specialist and Advanced Practice Skills

Introduction

The preceding chapters of this book have explored all the key components of the knowledge and competence that are required for effective practice teaching, namely the rationales and scope of this role, ways of establishing and managing working relationships within healthcare, facilitating the acquisition of generic, specialist and advanced clinical practice skills and knowledge, the practice teacher as an evidence-based practitioner and practice developer, an assessment of specialist and advanced practice knowledge and competence, and how the practice teacher exercises accountability and leadership.

Practice teaching in healthcare is a relatively recent concept and responsibility, with its aim being to facilitate learning and the assessment of specialist and advanced practice. Because of the protracted journey in defining and identifying the precise nature of specialist and advanced practice roles, there are features of the role that are still evolving, and unanticipated areas of development as well as aspects that might prove problematic might surface as the role gradually becomes more widely established in healthcare and social care.

This chapter identifies potential problematic areas in the practice teacher role, and further developments. Prominent issues identified in the analyses presented in the preceding chapters are explored in more detail, with a view to ascertaining the outcomes and possible solutions to them.

Chapter outcomes

On completion of this chapter you should be able to:

1   Identify the current structures and the likely problematic areas, issues and challenges related to the practice teacher role of specialist and advanced practitioners, and also the alternative career structures available to them.

2 Explain issues and developments related to facilitating the learning of evidence-based specialist and advanced practice knowledge and competence, and practice development, as well as issues in the professional education of healthcare professionals and students.

3 Demonstrate comprehension of the practice teacher's leadership in teaching and in assessing specialist and advanced practice knowledge and competence, and in confirmation and signing off practice proficiency, in the context of 'due regard'.

4 Evaluate developments in the educational preparation of practice teacher-cum-specialist or advanced practice roles, and post-qualifying CPD for practice teachers, annual updates and triennial reviews.

5 Present a critically analysed account of ways in which contemporary issues in practice teaching in healthcare and social care professions can be pre-empted or resolved.

Current structures for specialist and advanced practice, and the practice-teaching role

Changes in health service provision are continuous. They are based on numerous factors that impinge on various areas of the service, and on the ways in which they are provided. Changes that affect practice teaching, as well as specialist and advanced practice roles, are instigated by changes in society's healthcare needs, and by research, government policies and technological advances. Government policies also affect the career structure of qualified and experienced nurses. This section of the chapter explores key developments and issues related to specialist and advanced practice, the career structure of specialist and advanced practitioners, as features related to the practice teacher role.

Identifying issues related to specialist and advanced practice

There are a number of frameworks for systematically analysing novel or unclear concepts, such as practice teaching and advanced nursing practice, so as to identify the concept's strengths and likely problematic areas. They can be done through structured models of evaluation such as those identified in Chapter 7, after they have been implemented, or through such activities as SWOT, PESTLE or similar analyses.

Action point 8.1: Analysis of specialist and advanced practice

Draw the diagram that follows immediately on a sheet of paper, and complete the boxes in as much detail as you can on the topic of specialist and advanced practice. This exercise is more beneficially executed jointly by two healthcare professionals or as a group of specialist, advanced or senior practitioners.

(Continued)

(Continued)

PESTLE analysis of specialist and advanced practice

POLITICAL • European working time directive requirements •	EDUCATIONAL • Number of specialist or advanced practice nurses • .....
SOCIAL • Patients feel they can talk to nurses, ask them to explain what the doctor said •	TECHNOLOGICAL • Can utilise sophisticated devices that can lead to prompter and more efficient care • .....
LEGAL • Accountable for a greater range of activities •	ETHICAL • Physical, social and psychological benefits to the patient • .....

The above analysis can be utilised to deconstruct and clarify the practice teacher's specialist or advanced practitioner roles as emerging concepts at that point in time. You should have found this exercise useful, as for instance under 'technological' you might have mentioned the availability of novel medical technology, as well as the costs of purchasing and running them, and so on.

A more scientific way of systematically analysing a novel professional concept when the implications of the concept are as yet not fully clear, or if there is uncertainty about a concept, is through a concept analysis. Walker and Avant (2005) indicate that a concept analysis can be performed to determine systematically the structure and function of the concept, and subsequently to construct nursing theory. They therefore identify guidelines for doing so, which comprise:

- Select a concept
- Determine the aims or purpose of analysis
- Identify all uses of the concept that you can discover
- Determine the defining attributes
- Construct a model case
- Construct borderline and related cases
- Identify antecedents and consequences
- Define empirical referents (for critical attributes).

Concept analysis of a specific notion can enable identification of its various facets, following which the emerging theories can be scientifically tested using relevant research methods in the actual context in which they are meant to be applied, which also provides a means of triangulation to confirm and validate the theories. Risjord (2009) examines the uses of concept analyses in nursing, and concludes that this exercise is part of theory development, which can subsequently become practical theories in the subject area or field of practice. Risjord (2009), however, warns against the danger of generalising too readily from concept analyses without re-testing them in the context of their application. In the context of this book, concept analysis of practice teaching can therefore be performed with a view to supporting learning and assessment in different clinical specialisms.

So, systematic analyses of specialist and advanced practice roles can also reveal previously unidentified benefits and likely problematic areas. For instance, as noted in Chapter 1, there is currently a lack of agreement on the definitions of specialist and advanced practice roles, and yet there are numerous specialist or advanced practice posts providing highly beneficial clinical interventions in acute care, continuing care and primary care services.

The prospect is that ANP qualifications will become registerable qualifications on the NMC's professional register, but this is in abeyance pending further consultation and a government level directive on this (NMC, 2008a, 2008b). The number of different ANP qualifications is one of the issues that need resolving in that, for instance, there are five pathways for nursing careers development in *Modernising Nursing Careers* (DH, 2006a) and eight clinical pathways in the *High Quality Care For All* report (DH, 2008b).

Longley et al. (2007) report on an NMC commissioned investigation into nurse education, and note that it is influenced by various enduring paradoxes (which the Darzi report refers to as 'challenges'), such as an ageing population that needs longer-term care versus fewer individuals of working age to pay sufficient tax to fund healthcare, and an increased need for the prevention of ill-health versus more need to provide cures and palliative care. This and other reports suggest that advanced practice tends to refer to meeting the healthcare needs of patients and service users mainly in one of the five DH (2008a) pathways, and is characterised predominantly by clinical work that in turn requires a high degree of autonomy, critical thinking and the application of knowledge, and includes research, education and professional leadership. However, these also apply to most nurses, including specialist practitioners, although the latter seems to refer to specialisation in a set of skills.

Community-based specialist and advanced practitioners are likely to have a crucial role in specialist community centres (also referred to as polyclinics) as they become established more widely. These specialist centres, which are large health centres with GPs, diagnostic, preventive and interventional services, form a concept that is one of the recommendations of the Darzi report (DH, 2008b).

Comparisons have on occasion been made with regard to the cost-effectiveness of specialist and advanced practitioner roles, in that whether or not care and treatment delivered by specialist and advanced practitioners cost less than when performed by doctors, as generally doctors' salaries are higher than those of nurses. Griffith (2008) explored this point and concluded that a referral to ANP leads to increased consultation, more tests being ordered and more services mobilised, and therefore not costing any less overall. However, interventions by nurses lead to higher patient satisfaction and the likelihood of fuller recovery from the health problem.

One of the problematic areas related to specialist and advanced practice roles is resistance to these roles by medical staff, including junior doctors, who can resent their traditional roles now being performed by nurses, as noted in Chapter 1 (Corcoran, 2008; *Nursing Standard News*, 2008d). The study by Corcoran (2008) on specialist and advanced practice revealed that even nurses are hostile to specialist and advanced practitioners. This is because some nurses in generalist posts might see themselves as being deskilled as they have a reduced opportunity to participate in certain clinical interventions, because specialist or advanced practitioners, or nurse consultants, are called on to perform them as expanded, extended or specialised roles (e.g. Castledine, 2000).

Besides, employers in primary care seem uncertain about whether the practice teacher qualification is equivalent to the previous CPT qualification, as those who hold the CPT qualification are paid on a higher salary band than those who do not.

Furthermore, Coombes (2002) reported some years ago that many nurses taking an educational preparation for extended roles that enable them to specialise in clinical interventions have to pay the course fee themselves, but without any guarantee of receiving extra payments on completion of the preparation, and when the extended role has become part of their regular clinical activities.

On the other hand, some reports highlight the issue of NHS trusts reducing CNS posts in order to remain within their annual budgets (e.g. Harrison, 2006, Mooney, 2008a). If these roles are reduced, then the question arises as to which healthcare professionals will deliver the healthcare provision that specialist and advanced practitioners have been providing until then.

Developments in quantifying specialist and advanced practice activities

Other components that can impact on specialist and advanced practice are not necessarily issues, but developments and progress. For instance, although funding for the NHS is, and will probably always be, a point of debate to retain the principle of the NHS as 'free at the point of delivery'. Government announcements in 2009 included substantial extra funding for health problems such as dementia (e.g. Blakemore, 2009a) and strokes and diabetes, in which CNSs will have key roles.

Related to funding is the concept of identifying the effectiveness of specialist and advanced practice roles, which it is generally advocated, should be ascertained in the form of patient outcomes. The concept of patient outcomes is still developing and clear definitions of the term have yet to be agreed.

Developments in the identification of specialist and advanced practitioners' functions using the 'Pandora' computer database were mentioned in Chapter 1. Leary et al. (2008) explored the dimensions of CNS roles in the UK using Pandora, and recorded CNSs' activities as a series of events with eight dimensions to each event. The work of 463 CNSs over 2,778 days in England, Scotland and Wales from June 2006 to September 2008 was recorded, including clinical work, such as physical assessment, referral, symptom control and 'rescue' work, as well as administration (with about half of these administrative tasks identified as being suitable for secretarial staff to undertake). Research, education and consultation accounted for less time. However, Leary et al. conclude that CNSs in this study spent much of their time doing complex clinical work, including that done over the telephone.

Such work by CNSs takes place in many different contexts using a wide range of interventions that are diverse, which make comparisons difficult because CNSs themselves find it difficult to articulate their contribution to patient and service-user care as specialists. More research is recommended to ascertain quality, safety and efficiency in CNS roles.

Current developments also include developing national 'metrics' as the new quality indicators designed to measure the nature and impact of nursing interventions as a quality assurance mechanism. Metrics was identified in the Darzi *High Quality Care For All* report (DH, 2008b), and a report by the King's College London National Nursing Research Unit (Griffiths, 2008), which was commissioned by the Department of Health to support the nursing contribution as outcome indicators for nursing and the evidence base for nursing interventions. The latter concludes by making a number of recommendations including identifying the 'best bets' for current posts and future developments.

Mooney (2009b) reports on emerging evidence of the effect of this enterprise as 'assessment metrics' cuts falls by 26 per cent in older adults. An alternative to metrics is the developing 'Nursing Work Index Revised' model of measuring nursing practice (e.g. Slater and McCormack, 2007).

However, in contrast to the empirical precision being sought by Pandora and metrics enterprises, is the use of intuition by 'expert' nurses. Benner (2001) is one of several researchers whose qualitative enquiries conclude that expert nurses in particular tend to use their intuition as well as hard data in making decisions related to assessment of patients' and service users' health problems and clinical interventions. However, intuition appears to be in sharp contrast to the routinisation and normalisation of EBP in clinical practice, as also noted by Traynor (2009). So although intuition appears to have a definite place in clinical interventions, it is a mental activity by healthcare professionals, which is related to perception and intelligence, and which therefore needs deciphering.

Up-to-date developments, including those based on research on CNS and ANP roles, are regularly published in specialism-specific journals such as *Emergency Nurse, Community Practitioner,* and also in more generic international specialist and advanced practice journals such as *Clinical Nurse Specialist* and *Journal of Advanced Nursing.*

Career structure of specialist and advanced practitioners

There are aspects of the practice teacher role whose development and definition are contingent upon national-level policy decisions, including whether and which specialist and advanced practice qualification should be recorded on the NMC's professional register, and developments related to the period of preceptorship advocated in the Darzi report (DH, 2008b).

Current developments in specialist and advanced practice are closely linked to the career structure of senior nurses which is being explored at national level through publications in influential government documents such as: (1) *Towards a Framework for Post-registration Nursing Careers – Consultation Response Report* (DH, 2008a); (2) the CNOs *'Modernising Nursing Careers'* (DH, 2006a); and (3) *High Quality Care For All – NHS Next Stage Review Final Report* (DH, 2008b). They are

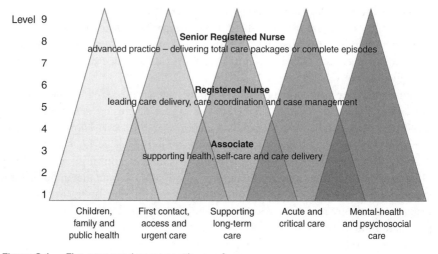

Figure 8.1   *Five proposed career pathways for nurses*
Source: (DH, 2008a)

closely linked to the nurse taking employment on gaining their nursing qualification, and the first above-mentioned document which is a '*consultation response report*' suggests five career pathways for nurses as identified in Figure 8.1. The consultation was triggered by the CNOs '*Modernising Nursing Careers*' (DH, 2006a) document. The *High Quality Care For All* document explored eight areas of care and treatment which can be perceived as areas of specialisation, and therefore the career paths of healthcare professionals.

A fourth highly influential sector, which is an offshoot of the Department of Health, is Skills for Health, who recently published a nine-level career and professional development framework for healthcare professionals, as noted in Box 1.2 in Chapter 1. Consequently, further discussion is afoot to decide on how many career pathways there should be, as some indicate that the five pathways will be too generalised, while others favour retaining four pathways in line with contemporary pre-registration branch programmes, and yet the Darzi report seems to suggest eight.

Decisions also need to be made as to whether nurses should join the proposed career pathway straight away after qualifying, or after a period of rotation in different specialist practice settings in the first year or two of their careers. There is also concern that the skills required in caring for service users with learning disabilities are not sufficiently recognised in the report, which can lead to a loss of specialist skills in this area. As yet unresolved areas also include matching job titles to academic levels of educational attainment, and for clarity in enabling those who want to change career pathway at some point in their careers to do so.

Current career progression seems to favour moving from registered practitioner to specialist practitioner, and then advanced practitioner, and later to the consultant nurse or equivalent position, and beyond.

Challenges of various practice teacher roles

The practice teaching role of the specialist or advanced practitioner can itself present challenges that the practice teacher has to try and anticipate, and then manage.

Action point 8.2: Roles of the practice teacher

As noted earlier in this book, practice teachers are registrants who are competent in the NMC outcomes for mentors, and who have subsequently gained further knowledge, skills and competence in both their specialist area of practice and in the NMC's stage 3 teaching role, and who facilitates learning, supervises and assesses students in the practice setting (NMC, 2008a). Consider the practice teacher's activities as detailed in this book, and identify what you consider to be the likely or actual issues related to this role. A SWOT analysis is one way of doing this.

SWOT analysis of practice teacher role

STRENGTHS	WEAKNESSES
• .... •	• .... • .....
THREATS	OPPORTUNITIES
• .... •	• .... • .....

As noted before, research on the practice teacher role within its current NMC definition is sparse. Bray and Nettleton (2007) report on a study that investigated nursing, medicine and midwifery mentors' and mentees' perceptions of the mentor's dual role as teacher as well as summative assessor of competence in specified skills, and the context within which the role is conducted. They found that there is 'role confusion' in professional education in that mentors struggle with this dual role, and there is conflict within this responsibility. The role of assessor is consequently poorly recognised and the complexity of being both an assessor and a supporter/friend can therefore be problematic because of the mutual teaching and learning relationship they form during the placement.

Recent research on students' perceptions of characteristics of mentors that can enable effective practice teaching includes Kelly's (2007) study which elicited specific characteristics – see Box 8.1. However, this study used a small sample of only 30 subjects, and although the findings seem logical and do contribute to existing knowledge in the field, they are not generalisable to all mentors.

Box 8.1   Students' perceptions of mentors' characteristics

KNOWLEDGE

- Clinical knowledge
- Pedagogical knowledge
- Content knowledge
- Knowledge of learner
- General knowledge
- Curriculum knowledge
- Knowing self
- Political knowledge

COMMUNICATION SKILLS

- Empathy
- Congruence
- Positive regard
- Listening
- Respectful/calm co-learner

FEEDBACK

- Positive feedback
- Negative feedback
- Private timely feedback
- Trust
- Honesty

ENVIRONMENTAL FACTORS

- Availability
- Acceptance by staff
- Climate
- Student–teacher ratios
- Peer support

Source: Kelly, 2007

Facilitating learning of evidence-based practice

As a specialist or advanced practitioner, the practice teacher's role includes ensuring that their clinical practice is evidence based, and that they develop their practice continually as required.

Evidence-based practice, research and practice development

Broadly, the concept EBP has become pretty universally accepted over time, and prevailing issues include ensuring that these concepts are not rhetorics but are at the forefront of daily clinical practice, and adequately supported by all necessary resources. Easier access to sources of best evidence, the capability to evaluate the nature of the evidence, the availability of necessary support with these and with practice development are some of the areas that can be problematic and must therefore be appropriately managed.

Regular post-implementation evaluation of the evidence is very important to monitoring its effectiveness, and also to check against any new evidence. However, as noted in Chapter 4, there are certain differences in EBP by different healthcare professions. For instance, EBM can be perceived as different from EBN in that EBM tends to focus primarily on physiological evidence and only minimally takes into account the effects of psychosocial factors on health, which are usually a feature of the holistic approach inherent within EBN. These can be perceived as either areas of conflict or as complementing each other.

Furthermore, practitioners need to be aware of levels of evidence in that if they feel that level 1 (systematically reviewed) evidence is not available, and that available is level 3, then they may decide to either conduct a closely monitored pilot run, or to implement the evidence as an empirical study using action research, or not accept the evidence at all.

Additionally, practice teachers are role models for healthcare profession students, and therefore they must be up to date with their knowledge and competence with regard to specialist or advanced practice themselves. As for practice development, innovation in healthcare is ongoing and relatively universal. As noted in Chapter 4, practice development is supported by guidelines issued by professional organisations such as the RCN (2007b) and live databases such as the Cochrane and JBI Libraries. Developments in EBP and practice development are regularly published in various healthcare journals, including specific ones such as *Evidence-based Nursing* and *Practice Development in Healthcare*.

Practice development is also supported by the government's Darzi report (DH, 2008b), particularly through recommending and supporting new care services by frontline healthcare staff, which is referred to as social enterprise. Blakemore (2009b) reports that the government is working towards offering cash prizes for innovations and entrepreneurial activities in patient care as one of the features of the Darzi report (DH, 2008b). However, entrepreneurial nurses (e.g. Mooney, 2009a) might find themselves in a position where they have to choose whether to become a non-NHS employee, or self-employed, when engaging in social enterprise.

Facilitating the acquisition of specialist and advanced practice competence

Issues related to the facilitation of learning tend to be localised. In general, students' (pre-registration and post-qualifying) academic and practice placement programmes are planned sufficiently in advance, and clinical settings are notified early of the start date of the practice placement, to enable adequate planning for successful placements (as also indicated by the NMC, 2008a). Every specialist and advanced practice student is allocated a named practice teacher prior to the commencement of supervised practice, and practice teachers should support only one specialist practice/SCPHN/ANP student at any point in time (NMC, 2008a).

Problematic areas could appear in relation to adequate protected time for practice teaching, and the availability of opportunities and students on specialist or advanced practice courses to teach and to assess their competence.

Planning the supervision of practice-based learning

Planning placements for specialist and advanced practice students constitutes a consideration of the student's individual learning needs and their course requirements. It is also to ensure they are fit for practice and fit for purpose by the end of the programme. Practice placements include a range of experiences, within associated trusts, and beyond. Nash et al. (2009: 48) report on a trial that aimed to enhance clinical placement for final-year nursing students, and found that 'one of the main beneficial aspects of the experience for students was the sense of belonging to a team that understood their learning needs and could work constructively with them'.

More comprehensive practice placement learning experiences can be usefully based on patient journeys and care pathways, and are referred to as learning pathways, which can in turn be based on the 'hub and spokes' model, as noted in Chapter 7. The level of student supervision by the practice teacher can vary from direct to indirect, depending upon the:

- nature of the activity the student is engaged in
- evidence of their current competence
- need to assess the achievement of NMC outcomes or competencies for progression on the programme.

Furthermore, placement learning constitutes 'work-based learning', several benefits and potentials of which, as well as related issues, are documented by Guile and Young (1996) and Moore and Bridger (2008), for instance, as noted in Chapter 3. This recent study also reported on a number of actual and potential problematic areas with WBL, and consequently made several recommendations, including:

- WBL must be embedded in individual 'performance and development review' mechanisms
- a pool of academic facilitators and mentors with experience of WBL should be identified to support WBL
- managers need to acknowledge and support WBL and provide protected learning time for this
- systems should be in place for problem solving and reflection.

Allocated learning time for practice teaching activity

Empirical studies such as those by Phillips et al. (2000) and Nettleton and Bray (2008) indicate that mentors struggle to find adequate time to fulfil their roles effectively, which they must do with minimal formal support from their work environment, in contrast to other professions. Practice teachers must therefore have time allocated to fulfil their roles, to reflect, give feedback and keep records of student achievements, especially in the final period of practice learning, to enable the practice teacher to fulfil this role more objectively.

The NMC (2008a) notes that practice teachers need to be able to commit themselves to supporting learning and assessment in practice, and therefore their workload needs to reflect the requirements of being a practice teacher. They require protected time, that is allocated time for initial, mid-placement and final interviews, for action planning and documentation, and for their teaching and assessing roles. They require time for the facilitation of learning and assessing proficiency at sign-off stages. The NMC (2008a) even indicates that practice teachers need time when undertaking work with a student, to be able to explain, question, assess performance and provide feedback to that student in a meaningful way.

Issues with the acquisition of professional competence

Professional competences of healthcare professionals are assessed in the context of 'standards of proficiency' which are already identified by the NMC, and which are then detailed as specific skills in the student's placement competencies booklet. The practice teacher's role includes an assessment of competencies and then making pass or fail decisions. In his research on knowledge and competence acquisition, Eraut (1994) explored how various professionals developed their necessary knowledge and competence, and noted that the term competence is not value neutral, as it can mean the ability to do something very well, or just adequately (i.e. not to the highest standard). Eraut also emphasised the need for evidence-based assessment when assessing professional competence, as does Gopee (2008b) in a more contemporary context, to ensure that assessments are valid, reliable and credible.

In healthcare professions the notions of competence and competency are explored quite extensively to ascertain their meanings and parameters. The NMC tends to identify competencies as practical clinical skills, whilst competence takes account of additional broader components including theoretical knowledge and attitude.

Bradshaw (1998) conducted an analytical review of the concept of 'competency' in an endeavour to define the term in the context of nursing, and identified 'uncertainty and fragmentation' in perceptions of the concepts. She indicated that this lack of clarity has implications for identifying competence at specialist and advanced practice levels of nursing practice as well.

Competence is identified by Benner (2001) in the context of two types of knowledge: practical knowledge (know-how) and theoretical knowledge (know-that). Cochrane et al. (2009) identify five dimensions of professional competence, which include knowledge as:

- cognitive competence (know-that, know-why)
- functional competence (skills or know-how)
- personal competence (know how to behave)
- ethical competence (possession of personal and professional values)
- meta-competence (cope with uncertainty, learning and reflection).

They note that activities associated with the term competence comprise different themes such as curriculum development, role profiles and self-appraisal, as well as the assessment of competence. This variety of perspectives on professional competence suggests that the meanings of the terms competence and competency are still evolving, and professionals involved in the assessment of students' competencies need to be aware of the dimensions of these terms which might yet be re-defined in the light of further research.

The practice teacher's leadership in the facilitation of learning and assessing competence

Facilitating learning for specialist and advanced practice, and for pre-registration finalist students, and an assessment of their knowledge and competence are obviously highly significant features of the practice teacher role. Some of the issues related to these and the practice teacher's leadership are also explored in this section of the chapter.

The practice teacher's leadership in facilitating learning

As detailed in Chapter 7, the practice teacher's leadership is an essential feature in both specialist and advanced practice, and in the facilitation of learning, and the latter includes creating suitable learning environments for students, and integrating theory and practice. However, in view of the findings of Philips et al's (2000), Duffy's (2004), Nettleton and Bray's (2008) and others' research studies that learning facilitators struggle to fulfil their variegated roles, which is further complicated by minimal formal support from their work environment, it is deemed important that practice teachers engage more proactively and methodically in forward planning for student placements. Forward planning entails careful time management and prioritisation to ensure that teaching and assessing roles are fulfilled effectively, as leadership also incorporates providing direction, and helping juniors and students realise their potential.

Leadership in the assessment of specialist and advanced practice knowledge and competence

Supervision and assessment by practice teachers has become mandatory since 2008 for students on ANP and SPQ programmes. The question, however, arises as to whether students on certain post-qualifying courses need to be assessed by practice teachers. Not all post-qualifying courses have a practice element, and some courses address only single clinical interventions (e.g. the prevention or treatment of leg ulcers), while longer courses address groups of health problems (e.g. circulatory disorders, tissue viability, or cognitive disorders). Students completing both types of learning beyond initial registration programmes can claim to have become specialist healthcare professionals, but not necessarily CNSs, as contemporary definitions of such senior roles are still in a state of flux.

Which courses constitute specialist practitioner courses, and whether students on them need to be assessed by a practice teacher, remain undetermined, and are identified locally. Consequently, students on single-intervention courses might not have to be assessed by a practice teacher, but by an appropriately experienced mentor. This situation could create confusion, but according to the NMC (2008a), students undertaking courses in 'learning beyond initial registration' can be assessed by a (sign-off) mentor (unless local commissioners and course leaders have specified jointly that this needs to be by a practice teacher). However, SCPHN students must be assessed by qualified practice teachers.

Confirmation of, and signing-off, practice proficiency

In their educational preparation programme for the role, or maybe in a previous programme, practice teachers will have been educationally prepared for assessing student performance in practice in programmes leading to registration on the NMC's professional register – as an SCPHN or an ANP. They will have explored their own accountability in relation to their decisions to pass, refer or fail individual students, based on their judgement of whether each student is capable of safe and effective practice for specific clinical interventions. Practice teachers will also be deemed to have met the NMC's additional criteria for signing-off proficiency at the end of an educational preparation programme.

Signing-off proficiency has been introduced for cohorts of pre-registration students who commenced on their educational preparation programmes in September 2007. The NMC indicates that, in the first instance, placement providers are required to identify sign-off mentors and practice teachers from those registrants who currently make judgements regarding students' capabilities for safe and effective practice for entry to the register. Trainee practice teachers do so by undertaking an NMC-approved preparation programme of being supervised on at least three occasions for signing-off proficiency at the end of a final placement by an existing sign-off mentor or practice teacher.

Practice teachers must also demonstrate 'due regard', whereby only a registered SCPHN in the same field of practice may sign-off an SCPHN student in that field of practice (NMC, 2008a). The NMC therefore indicates that the practice teacher is responsible and accountable for making the final signing off of proficiency, which then contributes to the portfolio of evidence considered by the university's Examination and Assessment Board, and confirms to the NMC that the proficiencies in relation to both theory and practice, as well as all other programme requirements, have been met fully by the student.

However, the non-availability of SCPHN, SPQ, ANP or pre-registration students in their area of practice can also present difficulties for trainee practice teachers if this constitutes limited opportunities for them to undertake the supervised signing off of students during the period of the preparation programme (normally six months), or even after.

Intra- and inter-practice teacher reliability in the assessment of competence

As identified over the years (e.g. ENB, 1997) an assessment of competence has to fulfil the essential criteria of validity and reliability, which is noted in Chapter 5. Accordingly, the practice teacher needs to self-evaluate regularly the extent to which they are meeting intra- and inter-practice teacher reliability. Reliability in assessments refers to ensuring that on a near-identical performance of a clinical skill, the assessee will be awarded the same result by the same and other practice teachers. The extent to which intra- and inter-practice teacher reliability is achieved can be ascertained by the practice teacher by continuous self-monitoring, discussion with members of the clinical team, and also in small groups at annual update workshops and study days.

Educational preparation and continuing professional development for practice teachers

After completing the educational preparation for the practice teacher role, it is up to individual healthcare professionals to monitor their own effectiveness as practice teachers, and engage in CPD related to specialist or advanced practice and sign-off proficiency status. Annual updates and triennial reviews, lifelong learning responsibilities and organisational learning are components that can facilitate this.

Effectiveness of educational preparation for practice teaching

As noted in Chapter 1, the practice teacher's educational preparation programme is planned by HEIs intending to offer the course, in collaboration with healthcare trusts' representatives, which then undergoes an approval event that is jointly led by selected incumbents from the university, external university assessors and the NMC.

The typical duration of practice teacher educational preparation programmes is of at least 200 hours of 'student effort' over a six-month duration. Demand for the number of practice teachers is expected to be low initially, but should increase because of the above-mentioned NMC requirement, and also if local healthcare education commissioners decide which SPQ and ANP course students should be supervised and assessed by appropriately educationally prepared practice teachers.

Generally, practice teacher courses are of shorter duration than the previous CPT and CPN supervisor courses, but then course participants are not required to have a mentor or assessor qualification beforehand, although desirable. This issue was also identified by Stevens (2003) who indicated that CPT courses were stopped as a result of the publication of *Standards for Preparation of Teachers of Nursing, Midwifery and Health Visiting* (UKCC, 2000). Stevens explored the need for the practice educator role in specialist community practice, and recommended that the practice educator role in the community to support students on specialist programmes should be strengthened.

This point was also highlighted in a study by Ewens et al. (2001) who explored whether specialist community nurse education prepares nurses for practice, that is to what extent it was 'fit for purpose'. They looked at the experiences of newly qualified community nurses, one year on in practice, which revealed that community nurses are very positive about their new role and their work with clients and patients, that they are able to use their newly acquired analytical skills in their practice, but feel inadequately prepared for the reality of the world of work, that is the pressure of work and the pace of activity in the health service. Ewens et al. recommended that curriculum planners should be aware of this and make appropriate adjustments in the programme, advisedly in partnership with local healthcare trusts.

For specialist cancer and palliative care, Rosser et al. (2004) evaluated a 12-month programme that was designed to support learning for qualified nurses who were new to their posts. A two-day workshop, action-learning groups and a structured facilitation of learning ('mentorship') by established specialists in the field were instituted. Rosser et al. found that the presence of a 'mentor' (now a practice teacher) was an important mechanism for becoming competent in this area of specialist practice, and that there were also further benefits in terms of service development.

Sims and Leonard (2004) report on an experimental inter-professional post-qualifying practice education programme which was offered even before the NMC adopted the practice teacher title in 2005. The programme was offered to qualified community nurses and social workers as part of post-graduate awards, which were supported by nursing and social-work professional bodies as well as the College of Occupational Therapy. Sims and Leonard report positive outcomes and their recommendations include:

- building in seminar groups with an inter-professional mix, but with an opportunity for uni-professional work
- tutorial support
- use of portfolios for the assessment of competence
- workshops for the students' practice assessors.

Uptake of these recommendations is likely to be quite good.

Monitoring own effectiveness, and continuing professional development as a practice teacher

To ensure practice teachers complete their educational preparation programme successfully they naturally need to heed the course requirements laid down by the university, and provide evidence of achievement of the NMC outcomes for practice teachers. The university expects an appropriate level of academic work that is consistent with the programme's year of study, be it at third-year undergraduate level or at post-graduate level, which are identified in both the assessment criteria, and also more universally by the QAA (2008b) descriptors, for instance (see Box 5.1).

Following a successful completion of the practice teacher educational preparation programme, it is mostly up to practice teachers to monitor their own effectiveness in this role. It is also up to them therefore to access updating study sessions, self-evaluate their own standards within this role, and also to access support and advice as and when these are needed.

Placement providers are responsible for ensuring that an up-to-date local register of practice teachers and mentors is maintained. All NMC-approved programmes are monitored regularly, which may involve NMC quality assurance agents' visits to examine evidence that the NMC programme requirements are being met. Data on the register of practice teachers and mentors are one way of providing evidence that there is a sufficient number of practice teachers to support students on specialist and advanced practice programmes leading to a recordable SPQ, SCPHN or ANP qualification, and that these are up to date.

As with most educational preparation programmes, although course attendees should be deemed competent and fit for practice by the end of the programme, as noted in Phillips et al.'s (2000) study, they may self-identify the need for ongoing support and CPD to ensure efficacy. The practice teacher has to be up to date not only with generalist and specialist or advanced clinical skills, but also with the curricular requirements of the students they teach and assess.

Continuing professional development can be voluntary or mandatory, and can be influenced by career policies and guidance such as those issued by the DH (2004a, 2006a, 2008a, 2008c). Gould et al. (2007) discuss the impact of the *NHS KSF* and its implications for CPD, for NHS managers and university departments delivering CPD for healthcare professionals. They suggest that the *NHS KSF* has the potential to increase the human resources management aspect of the clinical nurse manager's role, but could have legal implications if, for instance, practitioners perceive that their needs for CPD have been overlooked by their employers to the detriment of their career and pay aspirations. It also has implications for universities as providers of CPD as it requires closer liaison between education providers and trust staff who commission education and training.

However, problems do arise such as reports of the vast amount of funds being diverted from CPD budget allocations to other areas (e.g. Twedell, 2008), which led to a campaign against this activity by the *Nursing Times* over several weeks in 2008.

Preceptoring newly qualified practice teachers

In addition to the signing-off proficiency role towards pre-registration students, practice teachers also have a sign-off role towards SCPHN students, and SPQ students as determined locally. The NMC (2008a) indicates that once a practice teacher has completed their educational preparation programme, they may require a period of support from experienced practice teachers to enable them to consolidate their preparation for the role, which implies a period of preceptorship for the newly qualified practice teacher. Thereafter, the practice teacher can be supported through clinical supervision mechanisms.

The Darzi report (DH, 2008b) strongly recommends a structured period of post-qualifying preceptorship for all nurses as part of its focus on the quality of care and treatment. In particular, it explicitly supports strengthening preceptorship for newly qualified healthcare professionals with a three-fold investment in structured preceptorship provision, whilst the NMC considers making preceptorship mandatory. Consequently, healthcare trusts have created preceptorship co-ordinator type posts to implement the mechanism.

The practice teacher may also be required to act as a preceptor to new colleagues. The concept has been mooted for a number of years as consolidation and further development from their then level of recognised 'fitness for practice'. General guidelines for preceptorship are provided by the NMC (2006d) on areas such as:

- who preceptorship is for
- the role of the preceptor
- the role of the 'new registrant'
- the period of preceptorship
- the preparation for preceptors.

The question related to preceptorship that needs addressing is whether the preceptee will be assessed on a standard set of clinical skills, or locally determined skills at a healthcare trust or unit level. Furthermore, what will be the consequences of a nurse being awarded a fail on some of these skills? Additionally, Duffin (2009) and others believe that widely reported understaffing in practice settings can hamper the implementation of this recommendation.

Moreover, practice teachers also have to maintain and develop their knowledge and competence related to extended roles in their specialist area. Practice teachers should be prepared to demonstrate to their employers, and NMC quality-assurance agents, as appropriate, how they are doing this. Furthermore, practice teachers may not be able to maintain currency if finalist pre-registration students are not on practice placements at the practice teacher's practice base on an ongoing basis, for example primary care settings, for assessing and signing-off proficiency.

Annual updates and triennial reviews

After qualifying as a practice teacher, the healthcare professional must participate in annual updates and undergo a triennial review to maintain and further develop their knowledge, skills and competence (NMC, 2009e). These events should provide the practice teacher with sufficient formal and structured opportunities to become up to date with new developments, as well as to discuss issues and problems, and to explore solutions to them. It is advisable then to include 'critical incidents' in practice teaching and updating activities in personal and professional portfolios as evidence of continuing learning. The purpose of annual updating is to ensure that those who support learning in practice settings (NMC, 2009e):

- have current knowledge of NMC approved programmes.
- understand the implications of changes to NMC requirements
- understand issues relating to supporting students
- make valid and reliable assessments of competence and fitness for safe and effective practice.

Healthcare professionals who have previously completed a practice teacher (e.g. CPT) or an equivalent course can gain recognition of their knowledge and competence, and utilise updating opportunities as required individually. Local healthcare trusts may have a self-declaration mechanism covering all eight domains or 26 outcomes for practice teachers to complete so that they can remain on the local register of practice teachers.

Update workshops are also an opportunity to explore relatively less charted areas such as intra- and inter-practice teacher reliability, as well as conducting assessments in challenging circumstances. The NMC requires placement providers to make provisions for annual updating, and conduct triennial reviews. Evidence of updating should form a component of the triennial review, which placement providers are responsible for, to ensure that practice teachers continue to meet the NMC practice teacher requirements, and remain on the local healthcare trust's register.

Lifelong learning and learning organisations

Practice teachers as healthcare professionals continue learning and keep their knowledge and competence in both specialist or advanced practice and in practice teaching up to date through various means, namely formal, non-formal and informal learning (e.g. Gopee, 2002).

They have to meet the NMC's PREP requirements to remain on the register, and engage in lifelong learning. To ensure that lifelong learning occurs in reality as a vehicle for facilitating CPD in nursing, certain mechanisms need to be instituted specifically for this purpose. Some of the key organisational facilitators for achieving this include annual development and performance reviews, Workforce Development Confederations, professional self-regulation and Investors in People awards.

It seems that substantial informal learning occurs through work-based contacts with other healthcare professionals, staff, course peers, and in social interactions, which also constitute the notion of human and social capital. In a study exploring nurses' perceptions of lifelong learning, it emerged that in addition to the informal and non-organisational factors that enable an achievement of lifelong learning, there are various organisational mechanisms that also need to be instituted, and are therefore essential to enable nurses to initiate and continue professional learning (Gopee, 2005). The three-pronged framework for lifelong learning that comprises individual, social and organisational factors identified by Gopee ensued from a qualitative study, comprising semi-structured individual interviews and focus groups with RNs.

Conclusion

This chapter focussed on contemporary issues and developments in practice teaching in healthcare and social-care professions, and in specialist and advanced practice. Practice teaching is a relatively novel role, and potential problematic aspects were explored, so that they can be acted upon. It examined:

- The current structures for specialist and advanced practice, and for the practice teaching role, issues related to specialist and advanced practice such as the endeavour to quantify specialist and advanced practice activities, the career structure beyond initial registration and various challenges of practice teacher roles.
- Facilitating the learning of evidence- and research-based practice, and practice development, facilitating the acquisition of specialist and advanced practice competence, allocating time for practice teaching activity, planning the supervision of practice-based learning, issues related to the acquisition of professional competence.
- The practice teacher's leadership in teaching, assessing and confirming competence at the pre-registration signing-off practice proficiency stage, in the assessment of specialist and advanced practice knowledge and competence, and intra- and inter-practice teacher reliability in an assessment of competence.
- Educational preparation and CPD for practice teachers and their effectiveness, and annual updates, triennial reviews and lifelong learning responsibilities

Although healthcare and learning support activities are planned beforehand so that they are accomplished effectively and efficiently, novel situations, issues and developments will always surface as society itself evolves. It is important, therefore, for practice teachers to be aware of the likelihood of such eventualities, and to countenance and manage them appropriately as they arise.

Conclusion

To continue to support the learning and assessment of students on healthcare and social care courses and other learners, in time, you may wish to continue developing your competence as a mentor and practice teacher to further levels. This might include continuing as a practitioner/clinician in your own specialist field of care and having a role that incorporates continuing to support mentors and recently qualified practice teachers as well as facilitating and assessing learning.

Practice-based learning support roles includes that of PEFs. For this, or if you plan to pursue a more academic role as a university lecturer in health related subjects, then this can be achieved by studying on a programme such as the Post-Graduate Certificate in Education that has been jointly approved by the Higher Education Academy (HEA) and a profession's regulatory body (e.g. the NMC). For having successfully completed a practice teacher course, you might be awarded credit points, and therefore you might wish to pursue a Master's in education programme. Both PEF and nurse lecturer roles will enable you to continue to support learning and assessment for healthcare practitioner learners, ensuring that they are fit for practice, purpose and award. Whichever route you choose, remember your actions will contribute to the development of competence in those who follow, and these actions ultimately benefit the health and well-being of those who your students will care for.

Glossary

clinical nurse specialist A nurse who specialises in a specific field of practice, has successfully completed appropriate educational preparation for the role, and who exercises higher levels of judgement, discretion and decision-making in clinical care than at initial registration.

formative assessment Interim assessment of competence to determine learning needs.

formative evaluation Evaluation that is conducted continuously during a contracted period to ascertain how the delivery is being received.

formative feedback Feedback that students receive from their learning supervisor on their achievements and their learning needs on a continuous basis.

hub and spokes model A model of learning pathway for students, which is based on the various health professions that patients encounters in their journey through an illness.

learning supervisor The practice teaching learning supervisor is a registered nurse or midwife who has successfully completed an NMC-approved practice teacher preparation programme (or a comparable programme which has been accredited by an HEI as meeting the NMC standards), the relevant specialist or advanced practice qualification, and is registered with the NMC in the same area as the student-practice teacher and for nursing in the same field of practice (adult, mental health, learning disability or child), and whose name is recorded on the employing healthcare trust's database of practice teachers.

link teacher A university lecturer who is named as a university–cum–healthcare trust liaison person.

mentor A registrant who has met the outcomes of stage 2 and who facilitates learning, and supervises and assesses students in a practice setting.

performance criteria The step-by-step actions that a student is expected to take to perform a skill safely and effectively, and usually comprising the healthcare trust's approved procedure or clinical guidelines for the particular clinical intervention. It is tabulated in two columns as 'actions' and 'rationales'.

post-compulsory education Formal education for over 16-year-olds.

Practice education facilitator Also known as a practice educator, a registrant who has undertaken an NMC-approved teacher preparation programme, or the equivalent, and has successfully achieved the outcomes defined in stage 4 of the developmental framework, but is based in a healthcare trust, and whose role includes supporting mentors and practice teachers, and may include maintaining the local register of mentors.

practice teacher A clinical nurse specialist or advanced nurse practitioners who have successfully completed an additional programme of study in the facilitation of learning and an assessment of the clinical competence of students on learning beyond initial registration courses, as well as pre-registration students at the signing off proficiency stage of their programme.

programme A higher-education course comprising a number of modules, where-upon the credit points awarded can add up to qualifying for a certificate, diploma or degree.

sign-off mentor Mentors are required to meet specified criteria in order to be able to sign-off a student's practice proficiency at the end of an NMC approved programme. All midwife mentors and practice teachers will have met the require-ments through their preparation programme.

simulation Role play and other purpose designed scenarios that replicate real-life health problem situations for students to assess, plan and implement care, in prepa-ration for encountering actual real-life situations.

stakeholder A term that is used to identify all parties that have an interest in a spe-cific education programme, which is because the success or failure of the programme affects them in some way.

summative assessment Assessment of competencies with a view to awarding a pass or fail (as different from a formative assessment which aims to ascertain learn-ing needs).

summative evaluation Evaluation at a point in time when the views of the recipients of a unit of activity are summed up.

teacher (NMC recorded) A registrant who has undertaken an NMC-approved teacher preparation programme, or the equivalent, and has successfully achieved the outcomes defined in stage 4 of the developmental framework.

References

Adair, J. (1988) *Effective Leadership – How to Develop Leadership Skills*. London, Pan Books.

Agnew, T. (2005) Words of wisdom. *Nursing Standard*, 20 (6): 24–26.

Alimo-Metcalfe, B. (1996) Leaders or managers. *Nursing Management*, 3 (1): 22–24.

Anderson, L. and Krathwohl, D. (eds) (2001) *A Taxonomy for Learning, Teaching, and Assessing: A Revision of Bloom's Taxonomy of Educational Objectives* (2nd edn). New York, Merrill Press.

Anon. (2009) Review summaries. *Journal of Advanced Nursing*, 65 (1): 45–51 and 65 (2): 279–284. Available from: http://www3.interscience.wiley.com/journal/121575343/issue (accessed 3 February 2009).

Argyle, M. (1994) *The Psychology of Interpersonal Behaviour*. London, Penguin Books.

Arnold, E. and Boggs, K. U. (2003) *Interpersonal Relationships – Professional Communication Skills for Nurses*. Missouri, Saunders.

Association of Advanced Nursing Practice Educators (AANPE) (2009) *AANPE Terms of Reference*. Available from: http://www.aanpe.org/AANPEHome/tabid/448/language/en-US/Default.aspx (accessed 16 March 2009).

Bailey, M. E., Tuohy, D. (2009) Student nurses' experiences of using a learning contract as a method of assessment. *Nurse Education Today*, 29 (7): 758–762.

Baker, C., Pulling, C., McGraw, R., Dagnone, J. D., Hopkins-Rosseel, D. and Medves, J. (2008) Simulation in interprofessional education for patient-centred collaborative care. *Journal of Advanced Nursing*, 64 (4): 372–379.

Bandolier (2009) *What is a Systematic Review?* Available from: http://www.whatisseries.co.uk/whatis/pdfs/What_is_syst_rev.pdf. (accessed 31 August 2009).

Bandura, A. (1977) *Social Learning Theory*. Englewood Cliffs, NJ, Prentice Hall.

Barr, H., Freeth, D., Hammick, M., Koppel, I. and Reeves, S. (2005) *The Evidence Base & Recommendations for Interprofessional Education in Health and Social Care*. Available from: http://www.swap.ac.uk/docs/learning/Evidence08.doc (accessed 5 January 2007).

Barrett, D. (2007) The clinical role of nurse lecturers: past, present, and future. *Nurse Education Today*, 27 (5): 367–374.

Benner, P. (2001) *From Novice to Expert: Excellence and Power in Clinical Nursing Practice*. London/California, Addison-Wesley Publishing Company.

Biggs, J. and Tang, C. (2007) *Teaching for Quality Learning at University* (3rd edn). Berkshire, SRHE and Open University Press.

Blakemore, S. (2008) Nurse-led efficiency improvements increase time spent with patients. *Nursing Standard*, 23 (11): 10.

Blakemore, S. (2009a) Key role for nurse specialists in £150 million dementia strategy. *Nursing Standard*, 23 (23): 9.

Blakemore, S. (2009b) Government to offer cash prizes for innovations in patient care. *Nursing Standard*, 23 (21): 7.

Bloom, B. (1956) *Taxonomy of Educational Objectives: The Classification of Educational Goals, Handbook One: Cognitive Domain*. London: Longman.

Bondy, K. N. (1983) Criterion-referenced definitions for rating scales in clinical evaluation. *Journal of Nursing Education*, 22 (9): 376–382.

Boud, D., Keogh, R. and Walker, D. (eds) (1985) *Reflection: Turning Experience into Learning*. London: Kogan Page. [Reprinted 2002]

Bradshaw, A. (1998) Defining 'competency' in nursing (part II): an analytical review. *Journal of Clinical Nursing*, 7 (2): 103–111.

Brady, A. M. (2005) Assessment of learning with multiple-choice questions. *Nurse Education in Practice*, 5 (4): 238–242.

Bray, L. and Nettleton, P. (2007) Assessor or mentor? Role confusion in professional education. *Nurse Education Today*, 27 (8): 848–855.

Brennan, A. and Hutt, R. (2001) The challenges and conflicts of facilitating learning in practice: the experiences of two clinical nurse educators. *Nurse Education in Practice*, 1 (4): 181–188.

British Association for Counselling and Psychotherapy (2009) *Ethical Framework for Good Practice in Counselling and Psychotherapy* (revised edition). Available from: http://www.bacp.co.uk/admin/structure/files/pdf/566_ethical%20framework%20 revised%202009.pdf. (accessed 27 August 2009)

Brookes, D. (2007) Objective structured clinical examination assessment. *Nursing Times*, 103 (43): 30–31.

Brown, S. J. (2006) The experiences of lecturer practitioners in clinical practice. *Nurse Education Today*, 26 (7): 601–608.

Burnard, P. and Morrison, P. (1989) What is an interpersonally skilled person? A repertory grid account of professional nurse's views. *Nurse Education Today*, 9 (6): 384–391.

Burnard, P., Morrison, P. (2005) Nurses' perceptions of their interpersonal skills: a descriptive study using six category intervention analysis. *Nurse Education Today*, 25 (8): 612–617.

Burton, C. R., Bennett, B. and Gibbon, B. (2009) Embedding nursing and therapy consultantship: the case of stroke consultants. *Journal of Clinical Nursing*, 18 (2): 246–254.

Byrne, E. and Smyth, S. (2008) Lecturers' experiences and perspectives of using an objective structured clinical examination. *Nurse Education in Practice*, 8 (4): 283–289.

Callaghan, L. (2008) Advancing nursing practice: an idea whose time has come. *Journal of Clinical Nursing*, 7 (2): 205–213.

Canham, J. (1998) Educational clinical supervision: meeting the needs of specialist community practitioner students and professional practice. *Nurse Education Today*, 18 (5): 394–398.

Canham, J. (2001) The classification of specialist student practice: results of an exploratory study. *Nurse Education Today*, 21 (6): 487–495.

Canham, J. and Bennett, J. (2002) *Mentorship in Community Nursing: Challenges and Opportunities*. Oxford, Blackwell Science Ltd.

Care Services Improvement Partnership (2009) *Rapid Tranquillisation*. Available from: http://www.schizophreniaguidelines.co.uk/nice_implementation/rapid_tranquilisation/ (accessed 15 May 2009).

Cassidy, S. (2009) Using counselling skills to enhance the confidence of mentors' decision making when assessing pre-registration nursing students on the borderline of achievement in clinical practice. *Nurse Education in Practice*, 9 (5): 307–313.

Castledine, G. (2000) Are specialist nurses deskilling general nurses? *British Journal of Nursing*, 9 (11): 738.

Centre for the Advancement of Inter-Professional Education (CAIPE) (2007) *Creating an Inter-Professional Workforce: An Education and Training Framework for Health and Social Care in England*. Available from: http://www.caipe.org.uk/resources/creating-an-inter professional-workforce-framework/ (accessed 16 May 2009).

Clarke, J. B. (1999) Evidence-based practice: a retrograde step? The importance of pluralism in evidence generation for the practice of health care. *Journal of Clinical Nursing*, 8 (1): 89–94.

Clegg, A. (2000) Leadership: improving the quality of patient care. *Nursing Standard*, 14 (30): 43–45.

Clegg, A. and Bee, A. (2008) Community matrons: patients' and carers' views of a new service. *Nursing Standard*, 22 (47): 35–39.

Clifton, M., Dale, C. and Bradshaw, C. (2006) *The Impact and Effectiveness of Inter-Professional Education in Primary Care: An RCN literature review*. London, RCN.

Coady, E. (2003) Role models. *Nursing Management*, 10 (2): 18–21.

Cochrane, D., Palmer, J., Lindsay, G., Tolmie, E., Allan, D. and Currie, K. (2009) Formulating web-based educational needs assessment questionnaire from healthcare competencies. *Nurse Researcher*, 16 (2): 64–75.

Cochrane Collaboration (2009) *Cochrane Reviews – Alphabetically: [A]*. Available from: http://www.cochrane.org/reviews/en/index_list_a_reviews.html. (accessed 28 July 2009).

Comino, E. J. and Kemp, L. (2008) Research-related activities in community-based child health services. *Journal of Advanced Nursing*, 63 (3): 266–275.

Conway, J. (1996) *Nursing Expertise and Advanced Practice*. Dinton, Quay Books.

Cook, M. J. and Leathard, H. L. (2004) learning for clinical leadership. *Journal of Nursing Management*, 12 (6): 436–444.

Cooke, M. and Moyle, K. (2002) Students' evaluation of problem-based learning. *Nurse Education Today*, 22(4): 330–339.

Coombes, R. (2002) The advanced practice payment scandal. *Nursing Times*, 98 (49): 10–11.

Corcoran, J. (2008) *Senior and Advanced Practitioners as Part of the Multidisciplinary Team – The Reality of Practice* (RCN Nurse Practitioners conference, Liverpool). Available from: http://www.rcn.org.uk/development/communities/specialisms/nurse_practitioner/conference_presentations (accessed 20 February 2009).

Coster, S., Redfern, S., Wilson-Barnett, J., Evans, A., Peccei, R. and Guest, D. (2006) Impact of the role of nurse, midwife and health visitor consultant. *Journal of Advanced Nursing*, 55 (3): 352–363.

Council for Healthcare Regulatory Excellence (2008a) *About Us*. Available from: www.chre.org.uk/about/ (accessed 10 November 2008).

Council for Healthcare Regulatory Excellence (2008b) *Performance Review of Health Professions Regulators 2007/08 – Helping Regulation to Improve*. Available from: http://www.chre.org.uk/_img/pics/Perf_Rev_Report_1.pdf (accessed 10 November 2008).

Crawford, M. J., Dresen, S. E. and Tschikota, S. E. (2000) From 'getting to know you' to 'soloing': the preceptor–student relationship. *NTResearch*, 5 (1): 5–19.

Cross, K. D. (1996) An analysis of the concept facilitation. *Nurse Education Today*, 16 (5): 350–355.

Cullum, N., Ciliska, D., Haynes, R. B. and Marks, S. (2008) An introduction to evidence-based Nursing. In Cullum, N., Ciliska, D., Haynes, R. B., and Marks, S. (eds) *Evidence-based Nursing – An Introduction*. Oxford, Blackwell Publishing.

Cunningham, G. and Kitson, A. (2000) An evaluation of the RCN Clinical Leadership Development Programme. *Nursing Standard*, (part 1) 15 (12): 34–37 and (part 2) 15 (13): 34–40.

Curzon, L. B. (2003) *Teaching in Further Education* (6th edn). London, Continuum.

Darling, L. A. W. (1984) What do nurses want in a mentor? *Journal of Nursing Administration*, 14 (10): 42–44.

Davies, K. and Gilling, B. (1998) Building relationships. *Nursing Times Learning Curve*, 2 (5): 6.

Department of Health (1999) *Making a Difference*. London, DH.

Department of Heath (2000) *The NHS Plan: A Plan for Investment, a Plan for Reform*. London, The Stationery Office.

Department of Health (2001a) *Care Direct*. Available from: http://www.dh.gov.uk/en/Publicationsandstatistics/Publications/PublicationsPolicyAndGuidance/DH_4006865 (accessed 6 April 2009).

Department of Health (2001b) *National Service Framework for Older People that documents key standards for this age group*.

Department of Health (2001c) *Arrangements for Consultant Nurse Posts – for Staff Covered by the Professions Allied To Medicine PT 'A' Whitley council – Advance letter PAM (PTA) 2/2001*. Leeds, DH.

Department of Health (2002) *Developing Key Roles for Nurses and Midwives – a Guide for Managers*. Available from: http://www.dh.gov.uk/en/Publicationsandstatistics/Publications/PublicationsPolicyAndGuidance/DH_4009527(accessed 28 March 2009).

Department of Health (2004a) *The NHS Knowledge and Skills Framework (NHS KSF) and the Development Review Process*. Available from: http://www.dh.gov.uk/en/Publicationsandstatistics/Publications/PublicationsPolicyAndGuidance/DH_4090843 (accessed 6 April 2009).

Department of Health (2004b) *The NHS Improvement Plan: Putting People at the Heart of Public Services*. London, The Stationery Office.

Department of Health (2004c) *Patient Pathways*. Available from: http://www.dh.gov.uk/en/Healthcare/Primarycare/Treatmentcentres/DH_4097263 (accessed 6 April 2009).

Department of Health (2006a) *Modernising Nursing Careers: Setting the Direction*. London, The Stationery Office.

Department of Health (2006b) *Our Health, Our Care, Our Say: Making It Happen*. Available from: http://www.dh.gov.uk/en/Publicationsandstatistics/Publications/PublicationsPolicyAndGuidance/DH_4139925 (accessed 7 May 2009).

Department of Health (2006c) *Good Doctors, Safer Patients: Proposals to Strengthen the System to Assure and Improve the Performance of Doctors and to Protect the Safety of Patients*. Available from: http://www.dh.gov.uk/en/Publicationsandstatistics/Publications/PublicationsPolicyAndGuidance/DH_4137232 (accessed 27 December 2008).

Department of Health (2007a) *Trust, Assurance and Safety – the Regulation of Health Professionals in the 21st Century* White Paper. Available from: www.dh.gov.uk/PublicationsAndStatistics/ (accessed 11 March 2007).

Department of Health (2007b) *Guidance on the Single Assessment Process*. Available from:http://www.dh.gov.uk/en/SocialCare/Chargingandassessment/SingleAssessmentProcess/DH_079509#_1 (accessed 6 April 2009).

Department of Health (2007c) *Creating an Interprofessional Workforce: An Education and Training Framework for Health and Social Care in England*. Available from: www.dh.gov.uk/en/Publicationsandstatistics/Publications/PublicationsPolicyAndGuidance/DH_078592 (accessed 31 January 2009).

Department of Health (2007d) *Our Health, Our Care, Our Say – One Year On.* Available from: http://www.dh.gov.uk/en/Healthcare/Ourhealthourcareoursay/DH_073621 (accessed 8 February 2009).

Department of Health (2007e) *The Regulation of the Non-medical Healthcare Professions.* Available from: http://www.dh.gov.uk/en/Consultations/Responsestoconsultations/DH_066020 (accessed 27 December 2008).

Department of Health (2008a) *Towards a Framework for Post-registration Nursing Careers – Consultation Response Report.* Available from: www.dh.gov.uk/en/Consultations/Responsestoconsultations/DH_086465 (accessed 2 January 2009).

Department of Health (2008b) *High Quality Care for All – NHS Next Stage Review Final Report.* Available from: www.dh.gov.uk/en/Publicationsandstatistics/Publications/PublicationsPolicyAndGuidance/DH_085825 (accessed 10 July 2008).

Department of Health (2008c) *Delivering Care Closer to Home: Meeting the Challenge.* Available from: www.dh.gov.uk/en/Healthcare/Ourhealthourcareoursay/DH_4139717 (accessed 14 February 2009).

Department of Health (2008d) *The National Education and Competence Framework for Advanced Critical Care Practitioners.* Available from: http://www.dh.gov.uk/en/Publicationsandstatistics/Publications/PublicationsPolicyAndGuidance/DH_0840 11 (accessed 14 April 2009).

Department of Health (2008e) *Medical Revalidation – Principles and Next Steps – The Report of the Chief Medical Officer for England's Working Group.* Available from: http://www.dh.gov.uk/en/Publicationsandstatistics/Publications/PublicationsPolicyAndGu idance/DH_086430 (accessed 4 May 2009).

Department of Health (2008f) *Skills for Health Careers Framework Descriptors.* Available from: http://www.skillsforhealth.org.uk/js/uploaded/CF_%20Descriptors_jan_2008_3_5_GES_12.12.08.pdf (accessed 20 February 2009).

Department of Health (2008g) *Principles for Revalidation.* Available from: http://www.dh.gov.uk/en/Publicationsandstatistics/Publications/PublicationsPolicyAnd Guidance/DH_091111 (accessed 7 April 2009).

Department of Health (2009a) *European Working Time Directive.* Available from: http://www.dh.gov.uk/en/Publicationsandstatistics/Publications/PublicationsPoli cyAndGuidance/DH_093939 (accessed 24 April 2009).

Department of Health (2009b) *The Essence of Care.* Available from: http://www.dh.gov.uk/en/Publichealth/Patientsafety/Clinicalgovernance/DH_082929 (accessed 24 May 2009).

Department of Health (2009c) *18 Weeks Referral to Treatment Statistics.* www.dh.gov.uk/en/Publicationsandstatistics/Statistics/Performancedataandstatistics/18WeeksRe ferraltoTreatmentstatistics/index.htm (accessed 2 February 2009).

Department of Health (2009d) *The Design & Establishment of the Leadership Council.* Available from: http://www.dh.gov.uk/en/Publicationsandstatistics/Publications/DH_093342 (accessed 5 February 2009).

Department of Health and English National Board for Nursing, Midwifery and Health Visiting (2001) *Placements in Focus: Guidance for Education in Practice for Health Care Professions.* Available from: http://www.dh.gov.uk/en/Publicationsandstatistics/Publications/PublicationsPolicyAndGuidance/DH_4009511 (accessed 13 May 2009).

Dewar, B, J. and Walker, E. (1999) Experiential learning: issues for supervision. *Journal of Advanced Nursing,* 30 (6): 1459–67.

Disability Discrimination Act (1995) Available from: http://www.opsi.gov.uk/acts/acts1995/ukpga_19950050_en_1 (accessed 17 June 2009).

Disability Rights Commission Report (2007) Available from: http://www.direct.
gov.uk/en/DisabledPeople/RightsAndObligations/DisabilityRights/DG_400107
0 (accessed 17 June 2009).

Distler, J. W. (2007) Critical thinking and clinical competence: results of the implementation of student-centred teaching strategies in an advanced practice nurse curriculum. *Nurse Education in Practice*, 7 (1): 53–59.

Doel, M. and Shardlow, S. (2005) *Modern Social Work Practice: Teaching and Learning in
Practice Settings*. London, Ashgate Publishing.

Donabedian, A. (1988) The quality of care. How can it be assessed? *American Journal of
Public Health*, 260 (12): 1743.

Donaldson, J. H. and Carter, D. (2005) The value of role modelling: perceptions
of undergraduate and diploma nursing (adult) students. *Nurse Education in Practice*,
5 (6): 353–359.

Dowie, J. and Elstein, A. (eds) (1988) *Professional Judgement – A Reader in Clinical
Decision-making*. Cambridge, Cambridge University Press.

Drennan, V., Davis, K., Goodman, C., Humphrey, C., Locke, R., Mark, A., Murray, S.
and Traynor, M. (2007) Entrepreneurial nurses and midwives in the United
Kingdom: an integrative review. *Journal of Advanced Nursing*, 60 (5): 459–469.

Duffin, C. (2005) Pre-registration education to undergo major review *Nursing
Standard*, 19 (26): 4.

Duffin, C. (2009) Understaffing in threat to success of UK-wide preceptor scheme.
Nursing Standard, 23 (28): 10.

Duffy, K. (2004) *Mentors Need to Learn to Fail Students*. Available from: http://www.nmc-
uk.org (accessed 27th March 2009).

Embling, S. (2002) The effectiveness of cognitive behavioural therapy in depression.
Nursing Standard, 17 (14–15): 33–41.

English National Board for Nursing, Midwifery and Health Visiting (1991) *ENB
Framework for Continuing Professional Education for Nurses, Midwives & Health Visitors*.
London, ENB.

English National Board for Nursing, Midwifery and Health Visiting (1997) *Standards
for Approval of Higher Education Institutions and Programmes*. London, ENB.

English National Board for Nursing, Midwifery and Health Visiting (1999) *Evaluating the
Outcomes of Advanced Neonatal Nurse Practitioner Programme – ENB Research Highlights
No 36*. Available from: http://www.nmc-uk.org/aArticle.aspx?ArticleID=1695 (accessed
22 February 2009).

Eraut, M. (1994) *Developing Professional Knowledge and Competence*. London, Falmer Press.

Erikson, E. H. (1995) *Childhood and Society* (2nd edn). London, Vintage.

Ewens, A., Howkins, E. and McClure, L. (2001) Fit for purpose: does specialist community nurse education prepare nurses for practice? *Nurse Education Today*, 21 (2):
127–135.

Fava, G. A., Ruini, C., Rafanelli, C., Finos, L., Conti, S. and Grandi, S. (2004) *Six-Year
Outcome of Cognitive Behavior Therapy for Prevention of Recurrent Depression*. Available
from: http://ajp.psychiatryonline.org/cgi/content/abstract/161/10/1872 (accessed
20 April 2009).

Ferari, E. (2006) Academic education's contribution to the nurse–patient relationship.
Nursing Standard, 21 (10): 35–40.

Fernandez, R. S., Griffiths, R. and Ussia, C. (2006) *Effectiveness of Solutions, Techniques and
Pressure in Wound Cleansing*. Available from: http://www.joannabriggs.edu.au/pdf/
TR_2006_2_2.pdf (accessed 20 April 2009).

Flanagan, J., Baldwin, S. and Clarke, D. (2000) Work-based learning as a means of developing and assessing nursing competence. *Journal of Clinical Nursing*, 9 (3): 360–8.

Flemming, K. (2008) Asking answerable question. In Cullum, N., Ciliska, D., Haynes, R. B. and Marks, S. (eds) *Evidence-based Nursing – An Introduction*. Oxford, Blackwell Publishing.

Frankel, A. (2008) Analysing how senior nurses can become effective leaders. *Nursing Times*, 104 (35): 23–24.

Freeth, D., Reeves, S., Koppel, I., Hammick, M., Barr, H. (2005) *Evaluating Interprofessional Education: A Self-Help Guide*. Higher Education Academy Health Sciences and Practice Network, London.

Gagne, R. (1983) *The Conditions of Learning and Theory of Instruction* (4th edn). New York: Holt, Rinehart and Winston.

Gardner, G., Chang, A. and Duffield, C. (2007) Making nursing work: breaking through the role confusion of advanced practice nursing. *Journal of Advanced Nursing*, 57 (4): 382–391.

Garside, J., Nhemachena, J. Z., Williams, J., Topping, A. (2009) Repositioning assessment: giving students the 'choice' of assessment methods. *Nurse Education in Practice*, 9 (2): 141–148.

Gatfield, T., Alpert, F. (2002) The Supervisory Management Styles Model. In Goody, A., Herrington, J. and Northcote, M. *Proceedings of the 2002 Annual International Conference of The Higher Education Research and Development Society of Australasia (HERDSA)*. Available from: www.ecu.edu.au/conferences/herdsa/main/papers/proceedings.html (accessed 19 August 2008).

General Medical Council (2006) *Good Medical Practice*. Available from: http://www.gmc-uk.org/guidance/good_medical_practice/index.asp (accessed 17 June 2009).

General Medical Council (2008) *A–Z of ethical guidance*. Available from: http://www.gmc-uk.org/guidance/a_z_guidance/guidance_list/list_m.asp (accessed May 2009).

Ghazi, F. and Henshaw, L. (1998) How to keep student nurses motivated. *Nursing Standard*, 13 (8): 43–48.

Girot, E. A. and Rickaby, C. E. (2008) Education for new role development: the Community Matron in England. *Journal of Advanced Nursing*, 64 (1): 38–48.

Godson, N. P., Wilson, A. and Goodman, M. (2007) Evaluating student nurse learning in the clinical skills laboratory. *British Journal of Nursing*, 16 (15): 942–945.

Goldsmith, M., Stewart, L. and Ferguson, L. (2006) Peer learning partnership: an innovative strategy to enhance skill acquisition in nursing students. *Nurse Education Today* 26 (2): 123–130.

Goleman, D. (2000) 'Leadership that gets results'. *Harvard Business Review*, (March–April) 78 (2): 78–90.

Gopee, N. (2001) Nurses' perceptions of PREP. *Professional Nurse*, 16 (6): 1139.

Gopee, N. (2002) Human and social capital as facilitators of lifelong learning in nursing. *Nurse Education Today*, 22 (8): 608–616.

Gopee, N. (2005) Facilitating the implementation of lifelong learning in nursing. *British Journal of Nursing*, 14 (14): 761–767.

Gopee, N. (2008a) *Mentoring and Supervision in Healthcare*. London: Sage Publications.

Gopee, N. (2008b) Assessing student nurses' clinical skills: the ethical competence of mentors. *International Journal of Therapy and Rehabilitation*, 15 (9): 401–407.

Gopee, N. and Galloway, J. (2009) *Leadership and Management in Healthcare*. London, Sage Publications.

Gould, D., Berridge, E. and Kelly, D. (2007) The National Health Service Knowledge and Skills Framework and its implications for continuing professional development in nursing *Nurse Education Today*, 27 (1): 26–34.

Graham, I. D., Logan, J., Harrison, M., Straus, S. E., Tetroe, J., Caswell, W. and Robinson, N. (2006) Lost in knowledge translation: time for a map? *The Journal of Continuing Education in the Health Professions*, 26 (1): 13–24.

Graham, I. W. (1995) Reflective practice: using the action learning group mechanism. *Nurse Education Today*, 15 (1): 28–32.

Graham, I. W. and Partlow, C. (2004) Introducing and developing nurse leadership through a learning set approach. *Nurse Education Today*, 24 (6): 459–465.

Gray, J. A. M. (2001) *Evidence-Based Health Care. How to Make Policy and Management Decisions* (2nd edn). Edinburgh, Churchill Livingstone.

Griffith, H. (2008) What is Advanced Nursing Practice? In Hinchliff, S. and Rogers, R. (eds) *Competencies for Advanced Nursing Practice*. London, Hodder Arnold.

Griffiths, P./King's College London National Nursing Research Unit (2008) State of the art metrics for nursing: a rapid appraisal. Available from: http://www.kcl.ac.uk/schools/nursing/nnru/reviews/metrics.html (accessed 16 March 2009).

Griffiths, P., Renz, A. and Rafferty, A. M. (2008) *The Impact of Organisation and Management Factors on Infection Control in Hospitals: a Scoping Review.* Available from: www.nric.org.uk/IntegratedCRD.nsf/6f3dd209a0b87bb880256ff90033c2cc/a610 3999ac4f647f802574c700567bdb?OpenDocument (accessed 10 October 2008).

Guile, D. and Young, M. (1996) Further Professional Development and Further Education Teachers: Setting a New Agenda for Work-based Learning. In Woodward, I. *Continuing Professional Development: Issues in Design and Delivery*. London, Cassell.

Hamer, S. (2005) Evidence-based practice. In Hamer, S. and Collinson, G. *Achieving Evidence-based Practice* (6th edn). Edinburgh, Bailliere Tindall/Elsevier.

Hammick, M., Freeth, D., Koppel, I., Reeves, S. and Barr, H. (2008) A Best Evidence Systematic Review of Interprofessional Education BEME Guide no. 9. *Medical Teacher*, 29 (8): 735–751. Available from: www.google.co.uk/search?hl=en&ie=ISO-8859-1&q=hammick+IPE+2008&btnG=Google+Search&meta=cr%3Dcountry UK%7CcountryGB (accessed 20 Aug 2008).

Harrison, S. (2006) The tide has turned for specialists as trusts try to balance their books. *Nursing Standard*, 20 (39): 14–16.

Health Professions Council (2006) *Who Regulates Healthcare Professionals?* Available from: http://www.nmc-uk.org/aFrameDisplay.aspx?DocumentID=1809&Keyword= (accessed 9 February 2009).

Heron, J. (1989) *Six Category Intervention Analysis. Human Potential Research Project* (2nd edn). Guildford, University of Surrey.

Hichen, L. (2008) Matron accountability extended. *Nursing Times*, 104 (27): 7.

Higher Education Funding Council for England (HEFCE) (2005) *HEFCE Strategy for e-Learning*. Available from: http://www.hefce.ac.uk/learning/elearning/ (accessed 24 November 2008).

Huczynski, A. A. and Buchanan, D. A. (2007) *Organisational Behaviour: an Introductory Text*. (6th edn). London, Prentice Hall/Financial Times.

Humphreys, A., Johnson, S., Richardson, J., Stenhouse, E. and Watkins, M. (2007) A systematic review and meta-synthesis: evaluating the effectiveness of nurse, midwife/ allied health professional consultants. *Journal of Clinical Nursing*, 16 (10): 1792–1808.

Hundley, V., Milne, J. Leighton-Beck, L., Graham, W. and Fitzmaurice, A. (2000) Raising research awareness among midwives and nurses: does it work? *Journal of Advanced Nursing*, 31 (1): 78–88.

International Council of Nurses (2001) *Defining Advanced Practice*. Available from: www.advancedpractice.scot.nhs.uk/definitions/defining-advanced-practice.aspx (accessed 29 March 2009).

International Council of Nurses (2004) *Guidelines on the Nurse Entre/Intrapreneur Providing Nursing Service.* Available from: http://www.icn.ch/guideline_entreintra.pdf. (accessed 31 March 2009)

Jacobs, K. (2004) Accountability and clinical governance in nursing: a critical overview of the topic. In Tilley, S. and Watson, R. (eds) *Accountability in Nursing and Midwifery* (2nd edn). Oxford, Blackwell Publishing.

Jayasekara, R. (2008) Cognitive behavioral therapy for men who physically abuse their female partner – Joanna Briggs Institute, Adelaide, South Australia. *Journal of Advanced Nursing,* 64 (2): 129–130.

Joanna Briggs Institute (2008) *JBI Levels of Evidence.* Available from: http://www.joannabriggs.edu.au/pubs/approach.php (accessed 2 February 2009).

Johns, C. (1994) Nuances of reflection. *Journal of Clinical Nursing,* 3 (2): 71–75.

Jones, H. and Hardwick, S. (2007) Mentorship preparation for paramedic foundation degree. *Net2007 – 18th annual International Conference – Abstracts for Theme Papers, Symposia and Posters.* Available from: www.jillrogersassociates.co.uk/pdfs/Abstracts_booklet2007.pdf (accessed 4 October 2008).

Jowett, R. and McMullan, M. (2007) Learning in practice – practice educator role. *Nurse Education in Practice,* 7 (4): 266–271.

Joyce, B., Calhoun, E. Hopkins, D. (2009) *Models of Learning – Tools for Teaching* (2nd edn). Buckingham, Open University Press.

Kantek, F. and Gezer, N. (2009) Conflict in schools: student nurses' conflict management styles. *Nurse Education Today,* 29 (1): 100–107.

Kelly, C. (2007) Students' perceptions of effective clinical teaching revisited. *Nurse Education Today,* 27 (8): 885–992.

Kerry, T. and Mayes, A. S. (editors) (1995) *Issues in Mentoring.* London, Routledge and The Open University.

Khattab, A. D. and Rawlings, B. (2008) Use of a modified OSCE to assess nurse practitioner students. *British Journal of Nursing,* 17 (12): 754–759.

Kirkpatrick, D. L. and Kirkpatrick, J. D. (2005) *Evaluating Training Programs: The Four Levels* (3rd edn). San Francisco, CA: Berrett-Koehler Publishers.

Kitson, A. (1993) Accountability for quality. *Nursing Standard,* 8 (1): 4–6.

Kitson, A. (2009) The need for systems change: reflections on knowledge translation and organizational change. *Journal of Advanced Nursing,* 65 (1): 217–228.

Kitson, A., Harvey, G. and McCormack, B. (1998) Enabling the implementation of evidence based practice: a conceptual framework. *Quality in Health Care,* 7 (3): 149–158.

Koehn, M. L. and Lehman, K. (2008) Nurses' perceptions of evidence-based nursing practice. *Journal of Advanced Nursing,* 62 (2): 209–215.

Kolb, D. (1984) *Experiential Learning: Experience as the Source of Learning and Development.* London, Prentice-Hall.

Kouzes, M. and Posner, B. Z. (2007) *The Leadership Challenge* (4th edn). New York, Jossey-Bass.

Lankshear, A., Lowson, K., Harden, J., Lowson, P. and Saxby, R. C. (2008) Making patients safer: nurses' responses to patient safety alerts. *Journal of Advanced Nursing,* 63 (6): 567–575.

Large, S., Macleod, A., Cunningham, G. and Kitson, A. (2005) *A Multiple-case Study Evaluation of the RCN Clinical Leadership Programme in England.* London, RCN.

Le May, A. and Mulhall, A. and Alexander, C. (1998) Bridging the research–practice gap: exploring the research cultures of practitioners and managers. *Journal of Advanced Nursing,* 28 (2): 428–437.

Leary, A. (2007) Vital statistics: mathematical modelling can accurately demonstrate the financial benefits of clinical nurse specialists. *Nursing Standard*, 21 (17): 18–19.

Leary, A., Crouch, H., Lezard, A., Rawcliffe, C., Boden, L. and Richardson, A. (2008) Dimensions of clinical nurse specialist work in the UK. *Nursing Standard*, 23 (15–17): 40–44.

Levett-Jones, T., Lathlean, J., Higgins, I. and McMillan, M. (2009) Staff–student relationships and their impact on nursing students' belongingness and learning. *Journal of Advanced Nursing*, 65 (2): 316–324.

Lewis, F. and Batey, M.V. (1982) Clarifying autonomy and accountability in nursing services part 2. *Journal of Nursing Administration*, 12 (10): 10–15.

Lewis, R. and Noble, J. (eds) (2008) *Servant Leadership – Bringing the Spirit of Work to Work*. Gloucestershire, Management Books 2000 Ltd.

Liefer, D. (2005) My practice: government policy changes allowed an entrepreneurial nurse to pave the way for nurse-led general practices. *Nursing Standard*, 19 (22): 58.

Lipley, N. (2004) Two-year funding to train more leaders. *Nursing Management*, 11 (6): 4.

Lipp, A. (2007) Using systematic reviews. *Nursing Management*, 14 (7): 30–32.

Löfmark, A., Hansebo. G., Nilsson. M. and Törnkvist, L. (2008) Nursing students' views on learning opportunities in primary health care. *Nursing Standard*, 23 (13): 35–43.

Longley, M., Shaw, C. and Dolan, G. (2007) Nursing: *Towards 2015 – Alternative Scenarios for Healthcare, Nursing and Nurse Education in the UK in 2015*. Available from: www.nmc-uk.org/aFrameDisplay.aspx?DocumentID=3550 (accessed 31 August 2008).

Longley, M., Shaw, C. and Dolan, G./Nursing and Midwifery Council (2007) *Nursing: Towards 2015 – Alternative Scenarios for Healthcare, Nursing and Nurse Education in the UK in 2015*. Available from: http://www.nmc-uk.org/aFrameDisplay.aspx?DocumentID=3550&Keyword= (accessed 9 February 2009).

Lyons, E. M. (2008) Examining the effects of problem-based learning and NCLEX-RN scores on the critical thinking skills of associate degree nursing students in a southeastern community college. *International Journal of Nursing Education Scholarship*, 5 (1): 1–17 (article 21). Available from: http://www.bepress.com/ijnes/vol5/iss1/art21/ (accessed 13 April 2009).

Macnee, C. L. and McCabe, S. (2008) *Understanding Nursing Research; Reading and Using Research in Evidence-Based Practice* (2nd edn). Philadelphia, Lippincott Williams and Wilkins.

Major, D. (2005) OSCEs – seven years on the bandwagon: the progress of an objective structured clinical evaluation programme. *Nurse Education Today*, 25 (6): 442–454.

Manley, K. (1997) A conceptual framework for advanced practice: an action research project operationalizing an advanced practitioner/consultant nurse role. *Journal of Clinical Nursing*, 6 (3): 179–90.

Manley, K. (2000) Organisational culture and consultant nurse outcomes: part 2 nurse outcomes. *Nursing Standard*, 14 (37): 34–38.

Manley, K. (2008) Nursing talent. *Nursing Standard*, 22 (25): 18–19.

Manley, K., Hardy, S., Titchen, A., Garbett, R. and McCormack, B. (2005) *Changing Patients' Worlds through Nursing Practice Expertise*. Available from: http://www.rcn.org.uk/__data/assets/pdf_file/0005/78647/002512.pdf (accessed 5 April 2009).

Manning, A., Cronin, P., Monaghan, A. and Rawlings-Anderson, K. (2009) Supporting students in practice: an exploration of reflective groups as a means of support *Nurse Education in Practice*, 9 (3): 176–183.

Marlow, A., Spratt, C. and Reilly, A. (2008) Collaborative action learning: a professional development model for educational innovation in nursing. *Nurse Education in Practice*, 8 (3): 184–189.

Marton, F., Hounsell, D. and Entwistle, N. (eds) (1997) *The Experience of Learning* (2nd edn). Edinburgh, Scottish Academic Press.

Maughan, K. and Clarke, C. (2001) The effect of a clinical nurse specialist in gynaecological oncology on quality of life and sexuality. *Journal of Clinical Nursing*, 10 (2): 221–229.

May, C. (1990) Research on nurse–patient relationships: problems of theory, problems of practice. *Journal of Advanced Nursing*, 15 (3): 307–315.

McArthur, G. S. and Burns, I. (2008) An evaluation, at the 1-year stage, of a 3-year project to introduce practice education facilitators to NHS Tayside and Fife. *Nurse Education in Practice*, 8 (3): 149–155.

McCormack, B. (2009) Practice development: 'to be what we want to be'. *Journal of Clinical Nursing*, 18(2): 160–162.

McGarry, J. (2008) Exploring the nurse–patient relationship in the home. *Nursing Times*, 104 (28): 32–33.

McGaughey, J., Alderdice, F., Fowler, R., Kapila, A., Mayhew, A. and Moutray, M. (2007) *Outreach and Early Warning Systems (EWS) for the Prevention of Intensive Care Admission and Death of Critically Ill Adult Patients on General Hospital Wards*. Available from: http://www.mrw.interscience.wiley.com/cochrane/clsysrev/articles/CD005529/fram e.html (accessed 20 April 2009).

McGill, I. and Beatty, L. (2001) *Action Learning – A Guide for Professional, Management & Educational Development* (2nd edn). London, Kogan Page.

McGivney, V. (1990) *Access to Education for Non-participant Adults*. Leicester, National Institute for Adult Continuing Education.

McIntosh, J. and Tolson, D. (2009) Leadership as part of the nurse consultant role: banging the drum for patient care. *Journal of Clinical Nursing*, 18 (2): 219–227

McKenna, H.P., Ashton, S. and Keeney, S. (2004) Barriers to evidence-based practice in primary care. *Journal of Advanced Nursing*, 45 (2): 178–189.

McLellan, A. (2009) Recruit more health visitors now to help keep children safe. *Nursing Times*, 105 (5): 31.

McSherry, R. and Warr, J. (2008) *An Introduction to Practice Development in Health and Social Care*. Berkshire, Open University Press.

McVeigh, H. (2009) Factors influencing the utilisation of e-learning in post-registration nursing students. *Nurse Education Today*, 29 (1): 91–99.

Melnyk, B. and Fineout-Overholt, E. (2005) *Evidence-Based Practice in Nursing and Healthcare: A Guide to Best Practice*. Philadelphia, Lippincott, Williams and Wilkins.

Mezirow, J. (1981) A critical theory of adult learning and education. *Adult Education Quarterly*, 32 (1): 3–24.

Mintzberg, H. (1990) *The Nature of Managerial Work*. London, Prentice Hall.

Mitchell, K. R., Myser, C. and Kerridge, I. H. (1993) Assessing the clinical ethical competence of undergraduate medical students. *Journal of Medical Ethics*, 19 (4): 230–236.

Mockett, L., Horsfall, J. and O'Callaghan, W. (2006) Education leadership in the clinical health care setting: a framework for nursing education development. *Nurse Education in Practice*, 6 (6): 404–410.

Modernising Medical Careers (2009) *Speciality Training 2009*. Available from: http://www.mmc.nhs.uk/default.aspx?page=468 (accessed: 18 May 2009).

Mooney, H. (2008a) Specialist nurse posts under threat … but research proves role is cost-effective. *Nursing Times*, 104 (17): 3.

Mooney, H. (2008b) Judgement delivered on NMC. *Nursing Times*, 104 (25): 10–11.

Mooney, H. (2009a) 'Hostility' a deterrent to nurse entrepreneurs. *Nursing Times*, 105 (4): 1.

Mooney, H. (2009b) Assessment metric cuts falls by a quarter in pilot programme. *Nursing Times*, 105 (1): 2.

Moore, L. and Bridger, J. (2008) *A Realistic Longitudinal Evaluation of Work-based Learning of Qualified Nurses*. Bristol, University of the West of England and the Burdett Trust for Nursing.

Morris, J. and Maynard, V. (2009) The feasibility of introducing an evidence based practice cycle into a clinical area: an evaluation of process and outcome. *Nurse Education in Practice*, 9 (3): 190–198.

Moseley, L. G. and Davies, M. (2008) What do mentors find difficult? *Journal of Clinical Nursing*, 17 (12): 1627–1634

Moule, P., Wilford, A., Sales, R. and Lockyer, L. (2008) Student experiences and mentor views of the use of simulation for learning. *Nurse Education Today*, 28 (7): 790–797.

Mullins, L. J. (2007) *Management and Organisational Behaviour* (8th edn). London, Financial Times/Prentice Hall.

Nash, R., Lemcke, P. and Sacre, S. (2009) Enhancing transition: an enhanced model of clinical placement for final year nursing students. *Nurse Education Today*, 29 (1): 48–56.

National Committee of Inquiry into Higher Education (NCIHE) (1997) *Higher Education in the Learning Society (The Dearing Report)*. Norwich, HMSO.

National Institute for Health and Clinical Excellence (2009) *Press Release – NICE draft Recommendation on the Use of Drugs for Renal Cancer*. Available from: http://www.nice.org.uk/media/420/AD/2009009DraftNICEGuidanceDrugsRenalCancerv2.pdf (accessed 8 February 2009).

Nettleton, P. and Bray, L. (2008) Current mentorship schemes might be doing our students a disservice. *Nurse Education in Practice*, 8 (3): 205–212.

Numminen, O. H. and Leino-Kilpi, H. (2006) Nursing students' ethical decision-making: a review of literature. *Nurse Education Today*, 2 (7): 796–807.

Nursing and Midwifery Council (2004a) *Standards of Proficiency for Specialist Community Public Health Nurses*. Available from: http://www.nmc-uk.org/aDisplayDocument.aspx?documentID=324 (accessed 13 May 2009).

Nursing and Midwifery Council (2004b) *Standards of Proficiency for Pre-registration Nursing Education*. Available from: http://www.nmc-uk.org/aDisplayDocument.aspx?document ID=328 (accessed 4 May 2009).

Nursing and Midwifery Council (2005a) *NMC Approved Standard for Practice Teachers – NMC Circular 39/2005*. Available from: http://www.nmc-uk.org/aDisplayDocument. aspx?documentID=1178 (accessed 4 May 2009).

Nursing and Midwifery Council (2005b) *NMC Consultation on a Proposed Framework for the Standard for Post-registration Nursing – Final Report*. Available from: http://www.nmc-uk.org/aFrameDisplay.aspx?DocumentID=1004 (accessed 8 February 2009).

Nursing and Midwifery Council (2006a) *Mapping of the NMC Approved Competencies against the KSF Annexe 1 to NMC Circular C/05/160*. Available from: http://www.nmc-uk.org/aArticleSearch.aspx?SearchText=ksf (accessed 29 March 2009).

Nursing and Midwifery Council (2006b) *Responses to the NMC Consultation on Proposals Arising from a Review of Fitness for Practice at the Point of Registration – Final Report*. London, NMC.

Nursing and Midwifery Council (2006c) *Who Regulates Health and Social Care Professionals?* (available from http://www.nmc-uk.org/aFrameDisplay.aspx?DocumentID=1809& Keyword= (accessed 18 January 2009).

Nursing and Midwifery Council (2006d) *Preceptorship Guidelines NMC Circular 21/2006*. Available from: www.nmc-uk.org/aFrameDisplay.aspx?DocumentID=2088& Keyword. (accessed 9 June 2008).

Nursing and Midwifery Council (2007a) *Record keeping*. Available from: http://www.nmc-uk.org/aDisplayDocument.aspx?documentID=4008 (accessed 6 April 2009).

Nursing and Midwifery Council (2007b) *Sign-off status and Preceptorship for Practice Teacher students – NMC Circular 27/2007*. Available from: http://www.nmc-uk.org/aFrame Display.aspx?DocumentID=3261 (accessed 9 February 2009).

Nursing and Midwifery Council (2008a) *Standards to Support Learning and Assessment in Practice*. London, NMC.

Nursing and Midwifery Council (2008b) *The Proposed Framework for the Standard for Post-registration Nursing – February 2005 – modified March 2008*. Available from: http://www.nmc-uk.org/aArticle.aspx?ArticleID=82 (accessed 8 February 2009).

Nursing and Midwifery Council (2008c) *Good Health and Good Character Guidance for Educational Institutions*. Available from: http://www.nmc-uk.org/aDisplayDocument.aspx?DocumentID=4726 (accessed 13 April 2009).

Nursing and Midwifery Council (2008d) *The Code: Standards of Conduct, Performance and Ethics for Nurses and Midwives*. London, NMC.

Nursing and Midwifery Council (2008e) *Your Code of Conduct Applies to Your Personal Life*. Available from: www.nmc-uk.org/aArticle.aspx?ArticleID=3429 (accessed 21 December 2008).

Nursing and Midwifery Council (2008f) *Sanctions and Disposal Options* (available from: http://www.nmc-uk.org/aArticle.aspx?ArticleID=2390 (accessed 9 December 2008).

Nursing and Midwifery Council (2008g) *Meeting the Triennial Review Requirements for Midwife Sign-off Mentors who Support Midwives Undertaking the Standards for the Preparation and Practice of Supervisor of Midwives Programmes (NMC Circular 01/2008)*. Available from: www.nmc-uk.org/aDisplayDocument.aspx?documentID=3675 (accessed 8 March 2008).

Nursing and Midwifery Council (2009a) *The Practice Education Facilitator (PEF) Workshop: 29 April 2009*. Available from: http://www.nmc-uk.org/aArticle.aspx?ArticleID=3724 (accessed: 24 June 2009).

Nursing and Midwifery Council (2009b) *What Does a SCPHN Do?* Available from: www.nmc-uk.org/aArticle.aspx?ArticleID=2737 (accessed 20 August 2008).

Nursing and Midwifery Council (2009c) *Registration and Qualification Codes*. Available from: http://www.nmc-uk.org/aArticle.aspx?ArticleID=134 (accessed 13 April 2009).

Nursing and Midwifery Council (2009d) Record Keeping: Guidance for Nurses and Midwives. Available from http://www.nmc-uk.org/aDisplayDocument.aspx?DocumentID=6269 (accessed October 2009).

Nursing and Midwifery Council (2009e) *Additional Information to Support Implementation of NMC Standards to Support Learning and Assessment in Practice – published 10/02/2009*. Available from: http://www.nmc-uk.org/aDisplayDocument.aspx?documentID=5653 (accessed 25 June 2009).

Nursing Standard News (2008a) Be good role models, RCN congress to be told. *Nursing Standard*, 22 (24): 6.

Nursing Standard News (2008b) Judge calls for clarity from NMC after 'unsound' misconduct finding. *Nursing Standard*, 23 (10): 8.

Nursing Standard News (2008c) Diabetes specialist nurses could save the NHS £100m a year. *Nursing Standard*, 22 (27): 6.

Nursing Standard News (2008d) Nurse consultants blamed for junior doctors' lack of confidence and skills. *Nursing Standard*, 22 (46): 10.

Ousey, K. and Gallagher, P. (2007) The theory practice relationship in nursing: a debate. *Nurse Education in Practice*, 7 (4): 199–205.

Palfreyman, S., Tod, A. and Doyle, J. (2003) Comparing evidence-based practice of nurses and physiotherapists. *British Journal of Nursing,* 12 (4): 246–253.

Parish, C. (2006) Being nice is not enough for good leadership on the wards. *Nursing Standard*, 20 (41): 6.

Peplau, H. E. (1987) Interpersonal constructs for nursing practice. *Nurse Education Today*, 7 (5): 201–208.

Phillips, T., Schostak, J. and Tyler, J. (2000) *Practice and Assessment in Nursing and Midwifery: doing it for real (Researching Professional Education)*. London, ENB.

Pitts, J. Coles, C. and Thomas, P. (1999) Educational portfolios in the assessment of general practice trainers: reliability of assessors. *Medical Education* 33 (7): 515–520.

Price, B. (2005) Building a rapport with the learner. *Nursing Standard*, 19 (22).

Price, B. (2008) Enhancing skills to develop practice. *Nursing Standard*, 22 (25): 49–55.

Quality Assurance Agency for Higher Education (2001) *Benchmark Statements – Healthcare Programmes (Nursing)*. Available from: www.qaa.ac.uk/academicinfrastructure/benchmark/health/default.asp (accessed 12 November 2008).

Quality Assurance Agency for Higher Education (2006) *Guidelines for Preparing Programme Specifications*. Available from: www.qaa.ac.uk/academicinfrastructure/programSpec/guidelines06.pdf (accessed 12 November 2008).

Quality Assurance Agency for Higher Education (2008a) *Outcomes from Institutional Audit: Institutions' Support for e-learning*. Available from: www.qaa.ac.uk/news/media/pressReleases/26_Aug_08.asp (accessed 7 November 2008).

Quality Assurance Agency for Higher Education (2008b) *The Framework for Higher Education Qualifications in England, Wales and Northern Ireland* (2nd edn). Available from: www.qaa.ac.uk/academicinfrastructure/fheq/default.asp (accessed 11 October 2008).

Quinn, F. M. and Hughes, S. J. (2007) *Quinn's Principles and Practice of Nurse Education* (5th edn). Cheltenham, Nelson Thornes.

Raftery, J. P., Yao, G. L., Murchie, P., Campbell, N. C., Ritchie, L. D. (2005) Cost effectiveness of nurse led secondary prevention clinics for coronary heart disease in primary care: follow up of a randomised controlled trial. *BMJ*, 330 (7493): 707.

Ramsden, P. (2003) *Learning to Teach in Higher Education* (2nd edn). London, RoutledgeFalmer.

Redwood, S., Carr, E., Hancock, H., McSherry, R., Campbell, S. and Graham, I. (2007) Evaluating nurse consultants work through key informant perceptions. *Nursing Standard*, 21 (17): 35–40.

Reime, M. H., Harris, A., Aksnes, J. and Mikkelsen, J. (2008) The most successful method in teaching nursing students infection control – e-learning or lecture? *Nurse Education Today*, 28 (7): 798–806.

Renshaw, M., Hart, B., Harvey, M. and Harris, A. (1999) *Evaluating the Outcomes of Advanced Neonatal Nurse Practitioner Programmes (ENB Research Highlights 36)*. Available from: http://www.nmc–uk.org/aArticle.aspx?ArticleID=1691 (accessed 22 March 2009).

Risjord, M. (2009) Rethinking concept analysis. *Journal of Advanced Nursing*, 65 (3): 684–691.

Rogers, A. (2002) *Teaching Adults* (3rd edn). Buckingham, Open University Press.

Rogers, C., Freiberg, H. J. (1994) *Freedom to Learn* (3rd edn). Oxford, Maxwell Macmillan International.

Rogers, J. (2007) *Adults Learning* (5th edn). Berkshire, McGraw-Hill and Open University Press.

Ross, F. and Mackenzie, A. (1996) *Nursing in Primary Health Care – Policy and Practice.* London, Routledge.

Rosser, M., Rice, A. M., Campbell, H. and Jack, C. (2004) Evaluation of a mentorship programme for specialist practitioners. *Nurse Education Today*, 24 (8): 596–604.

Royal College of Nursing (2002) *Helping Students get the Best from their Practice Placements (a Royal College of Nursing Toolkit).* London, RCN.

Royal College of Nursing (2003) *Clinical Governance: an RCN Resource Guide.* Available from: http://www.rcn.org.uk/__data/assets/pdf_file/0011/78581/002036.pdf (accessed 13 February 2009).

Royal College of Nursing (2005) *Maxi Nurses, Advanced and Specialist Nursing Roles.* London, RCN – also available from: http://www.rcn.org.uk/__data/assets/pdf_file/0006/78657/002756.pdf (accessed 19 March 2009).

Royal College of Nursing (2006) *Nurse Practitioners 2006 – The Results of a Survey of Nurse Practitioners Conducted on behalf of the RCN Nurse Practitioner Association.* Available from: www.rcn.org.uk/search?mode=results&current_result_page=1&results_per_page=15&queries_search_query=nurse+practitioners (accessed 31 December 2008).

Royal College of Nursing (2007a) *The Impact and Effectiveness of Inter-professional Education in Primary Care – A RCN Literature Review.* Available from: http://www.rcn.org.uk/search?queries_search_query=The+Impact+and+effectiveness+of+inter-professional+education+in+primary+care (accessed 18 May 2009).

Royal College of Nursing (2007b) *Nurse Entrepreneurs – Turning Initiative into Independence.* London, RCN.

Royal College of Nursing (2007c) *Guidance for Mentors of Nursing Students and Midwives: an RCN Toolkit.* London, RCN.

Royal College of Nursing (2008) *RCN Competencies: Advanced nurse practitioners – an RCN Guide to the Advanced Nurse Practitioner Role, Competencies and Programme Accreditation.* Available from: www.rcn.org.uk/__data/assets/pdf_file/0003/146478/003207.pdf (accessed 31 December 2008).

Rush, B., Barker, J. H. (2006) Involving mental health service users in nurse education through enquiry-based learning. *Nurse Education in Practice*, 6 (5): 254–260.

Ryan, B. (2008) Positive partnerships. *Nursing Standard*, 22 (46): 62.

Rycroft-Malone, J. (2009) Institutionalizing evidence-based nursing practice: an organizational case study using a model of strategic change. *The 2009 RCN International Nursing Research Conference – Book of Abstracts page 112.* Available from: http://www.rcn.org.uk/development/researchanddevelopment/rs/research2009 (accessed 28 March 2009).

Sackett, D. L., Rosenburg, W., Gray, J. M., Haynes, R. B. and Richardson, S. W. (1996) Evidence-based medicine: what it is and what it isn't. *BMJ* 312 (7023): 71–72.

Satchell, G. (2008) *Hero Helps Others Fight for Cancer Drug BBC Breakfast report.* Available from: http://news.bbc.co.uk/1/hi/programmes/breakfast/7398632.stm (accessed 3 November 2008).

Savage, J. and Moore, L. (2004) *Interpreting Accountability.* London, RCN.

Scott, K. and McSherry, R. (2009) Evidence-based nursing: clarifying the concepts for nurses in practice. *Journal of Clinical Nursing*, 18 (8): 1085–1095.

Scottish Government (2008) *Supporting the Development of Advanced Nursing Practice – a Toolkit Approach.* Available from: http://www.advancedpractice.scot.nhs.uk/definitions/achieving-consensus.aspx (accessed 7 February 2009).

Secomb, J. (2008) A systematic review of peer teaching and learning in clinical education. *Journal of Clinical Nursing*, 17 (6): 703–716.

Sims, D. and Leonard, K. (2004) Inter-professional practice education. In Glen, S. and Leiba, T. (eds) *Inter-professional Post-qualifying Education for Nurses*. Hampshire, Palgrave Macmillan.

Skills for Health (2009a) *Key Elements of the Career Framework*. Available from: http://www.skillsforhealth.org.uk/careers-individual-skills-development/career-pathways/~/media/Resource-Library/PDF/Career_framework_key_elements.ashx (accessed 4 September 2009).

Skills for Health (2009b) *EQuIP – Enhancing Quality in Partnership Healthcare Education QA Framework*. Available from: http://www.skillsforhealth.org.uk/uploads/page/253/uploadablefile.pdf (accessed 22 May 2009).

Slater, P. and McCormack, B. (2007) An exploration of the factor structure of the nursing work index. *Worldviews on Evidence-based Nursing*, 4 (1): 30–39.

Smits, P. B. A., Verbeek, J. H. A. M. and de Buisonjé, C. D. (2002) Problem-based learning in continuing medical education: a review of controlled evaluation studies. *BMJ*, 324 (7330): 153–156.

Speers, J. (2008) Service user involvement in the assessment of a practice competency in mental health nursing – stakeholders' views and recommendations. *Nurse Education in Practice*, 8 (2): 112–119.

Spence, W. and El-Ansari, W. (2004) Portfolio assessment: practice teachers' early experience. *Nurse Education Today*, 24 (5): 388–401.

Sporrong, S. K., Arnetz, B., Hansson, M. G., Westerholm, P. and Hoglund, A. T. (2007) Developing ethical competence in health care organizations. *Nursing Ethics*, 14 (6): 825–837.

Steinaker, N. W. and Bell, M. R. (1979) *The Experiential Learning – A New Approach to Teaching and Learning*. New York, Academic Press.

Stevens, D. (2003) The practice educator in specialist community practice. *Journal of Community Nursing*, 17 (2): 30–31.

Sullivan, E. J. and Decker, P. J. (2009) *Effective Leadership and Management in Nursing* (7th edn). New Jersey, Pearson Education.

Tee, S. R. and Jowett, R. M. (2009) Achieving fitness for practice: contributing to public and patient protection in nurse education. *Nurse Education Today*, 29 (4): 439–447.

Thiroux, J. and Krasemann, K. (2007) *Ethics, Theory and Practice* (9th edn). New Jersey, Pearson & Prentice Hall.

Thorne, S. E. (2006) Nursing education: key issues for the 21st century. *Nurse Education Today*, 26 (8): 614–621.

Tilley, S. and Watson, R. (editors) (2004) *Accountability in Nursing and Midwifery*. Oxford, Blackwell Science Ltd.

Traynor, M. (2009) Intuition and evidence: Findings from focus group research into nurses and decision-making. Paper presented at the 2009 RCN International Nursing Research Conference – Abstracts p. 112. Available from: http://www.rcn.org.uk/__data/assets/pdf_file/0008/236699/2009researchbookofabstracts.pdf (accessed 25 June 2009).

Trudigan, J. (2000) The role of the clinical practice educator in tissue viability nursing. *Nursing Standard*, 15 (11): 54–62.

Twedell, L. (2008) SHAs divert training funds again. *Nursing Times*, 104 (11): 3.

United Kingdom Central Council for Nursing, Midwifery and Health Visiting (2000) *Standards for the Preparation of Teachers of Nursing, Midwifery and Health Visiting*. London, UKCC.

University of Surrey (2008) *Module Catalogue – Ethics*. Available from: http://www2. surrey.ac.uk/search/?cx=004166461246994000727%3Ap3yvcjwjr3o&cof=FORID %3A11&ie=UTF-8&q=accountability#1482 (accessed 2 December 2008).

Wakefield, A. B., Carlisle, C., Hall, A. G. and Attree, M. J. (2008) The expectations and experiences of blended learning approaches to patient safety education. *Nurse Education in Practice*, 8 (1): 54-61.

Walker, J., Crawford, J. and Parker, J. (2008) *Practice Education in Social Work: A Handbook for Practice Teachers*, Assessors and Educators. Exeter, Learning Matters Ltd.

Walker, L. O. and Avant, K. C. (2005) *Strategies for Theory Construction in Nursing* (4th edn). Upper Saddle River, New Jersey, Pearson and Prentice Hall.

Waters, A. (2007) Pandora maps the complexity of what clinical nurse specialists actually do. *Nursing Standard*, 22 (10): 14–15.

Waters, A. (2008) More than a nurse. *Nursing Standard*, 22 (46): 19–21.

Watson, R. (2004) Accountability and clinical governance. In Tilley, S. and Watson, R. (eds) *Accountability in Nursing and Midwifery* (2nd edn). Oxford, Blackwell Publishing.

Webb, C. and Shakespeare, P. (2007) Judgements about mentoring relationships in nurse education. *Nurse Education Today*, 28 (5): 563–571.

White, J. (2007) Supporting nursing students with dyslexia in clinical practice. *Nursing Standard*, 21 (19): 35–42.

Wilkes, Z. (2006) The student–mentor relationship: a review of literature. *Nursing Standard*, 20 (37): 42–47.

Williams, M. (2003) Assessment of portfolios in professional education. *Nursing Standard*, 18 (8): 33–37.

Williams, S. M. and Beattie, H. J. (2008) Problem–based learning in the clinical setting – a systematic review. *Nurse Education Today*, 28 (2): 146–154.

Xiao, L. D. (2008) An understanding of nurse educators' leadership behaviours in implementing mandatory continuing nursing education in China. *Nurse Education in Practice*, 8 (5): 312–7.

Xyrichis, A. and Ream, E. (2008) Teamwork: a concept analysis. *Journal of Advanced Nursing*, 61 (2): 232–241.

Index